Dentistry for Kids
Rethinking Your Daily Practice

Dedication

I would like to dedicate this book to Dr Christiane Gleissner. She was the first and only one who read the complete and raw manuscript, dedicating many hours while contributing some important suggestions from the viewpoint of a general dentist. She always motivated me and dispelled doubts. She will forever be an inspiration for me. May she rest in peace.

Library of Congress Cataloging-in-Publication Data

Names: Uhlmann, Ulrike, 1986- author.
Title: Dentistry for kids : rethinking your daily practice / Ulrike
    Uhlmann.
Other titles: Kinderzahnheilkunde. English
Description: Batavia, IL : Quintessence Publishing Co, Inc, [2020] |
    Translation of: Kinderzahnheilkunde : Grundlagen für die tägliche
    Praxis / Ulrike Uhlmann. [2019]. | Includes bibliographical references
    and index. | Summary: "This book offers professional and practical tips
    on communicating with parents and sets out to illustrate the
    responsibility involved in treating children"-- Provided by publisher.
Identifiers: LCCN 2020007937 | ISBN 9781647240134 (hardcover)
Subjects: MESH: Dental Care for Children | Child | Infant | Oral Hygiene |
    Dentist-Patient Relations | Pediatric Dentistry--methods
Classification: LCC RK63 | NLM WU 480 | DDC 617.60083--dc23
LC record available at https://lccn.loc.gov/2020007937

This book was originally published in German under the title *Kinderzahnheilkunde: Grundlagen für die tägliche Praxis* by Quintessenz Verlag (Berlin) in 2019.

QUINTESSENCE PUBLISHING
USA

© 2020 Quintessence Publishing Co, Inc

Quintessence Publishing Co, Inc
411 N Raddant Road
Batavia, IL 60510
www.quintpub.com

5 4 3 2 1

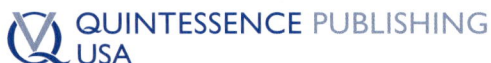

Editors: Leah Huffman and Samantha Smith
Design: Sue Zubek
Production: Sarah Minor

Printed in the United States

DENTISTRY
FOR KIDS
Rethinking Your Daily Practice

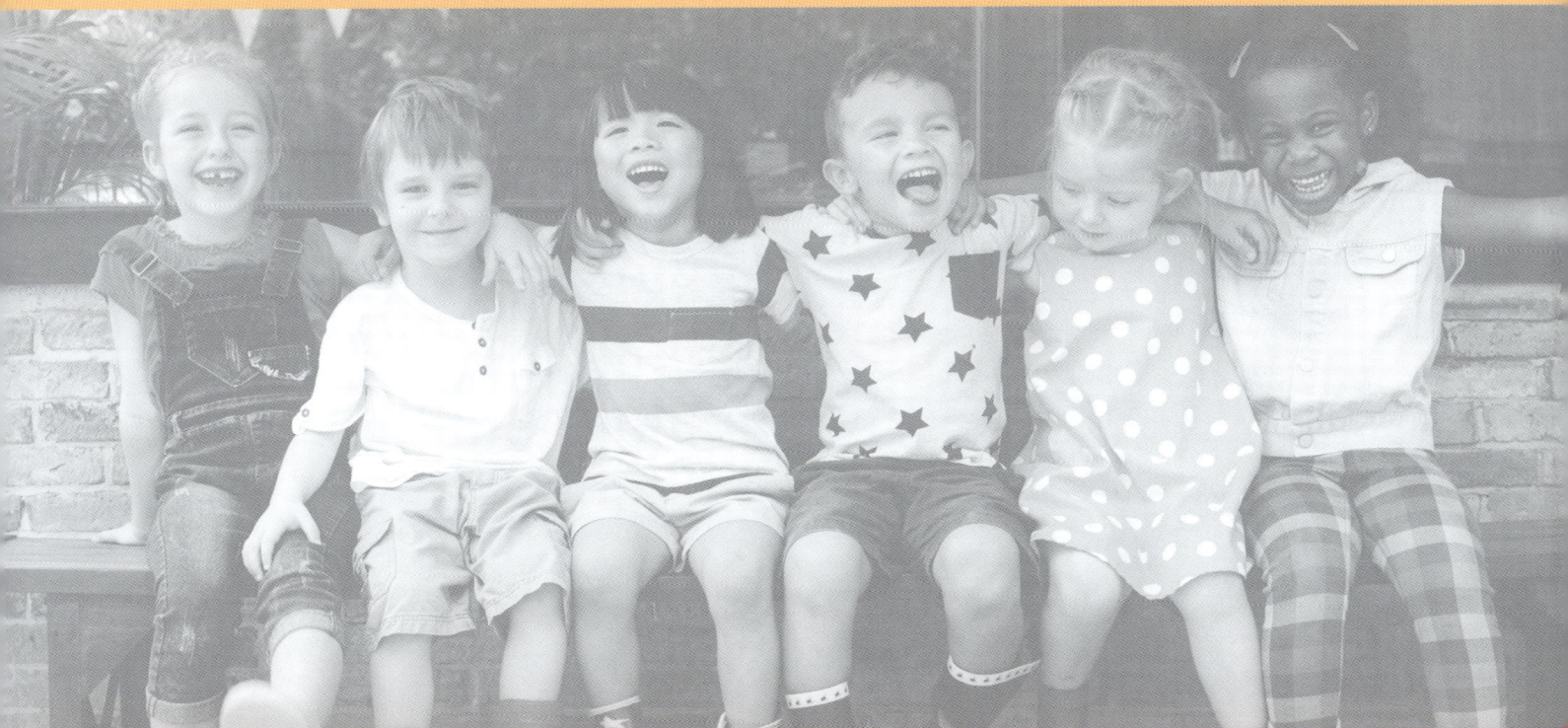

Ulrike Uhlmann, Dr med dent
Group Practice in Pediatric and Adolescent Dentistry
Leipzig, Germany

QUINTESSENCE PUBLISHING

Berlin | Chicago | Tokyo
Barcelona | London | Milan | Mexico City | Moscow | Paris | Prague | Seoul | Warsaw
Beijing | Istanbul | Sao Paulo | Zagreb

ABOUT THE AUTHOR

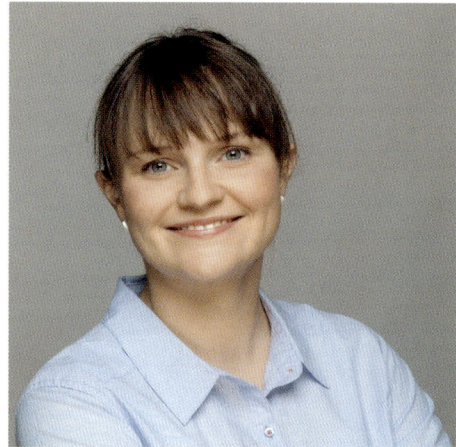

Ulrike Uhlmann studied dentistry at Leipzig University from 2005 to 2010. Even during her studies she showed a keen interest in children's dentistry. After her examinations in 2010, she worked in Halle/Saale for 4 years, during which time she learned about and came to love the whole gamut of pediatric dentistry. Interdisciplinary work with midwives, pediatricians, and speech therapists was and is a cornerstone of her professional ethos. At present she works on the staff of a family dental practice in Leipzig. As a speaker, she is also involved in the continuing professional development of midwives, speech therapists, educators, and other related professional groups in the field of pediatric dentistry. Together with a Leipzig midwives practice, she has also launched a parents workshop where relevant topics concerning children's oral health are explained to pregnant women and parents, raising their awareness. She is married and has four children.

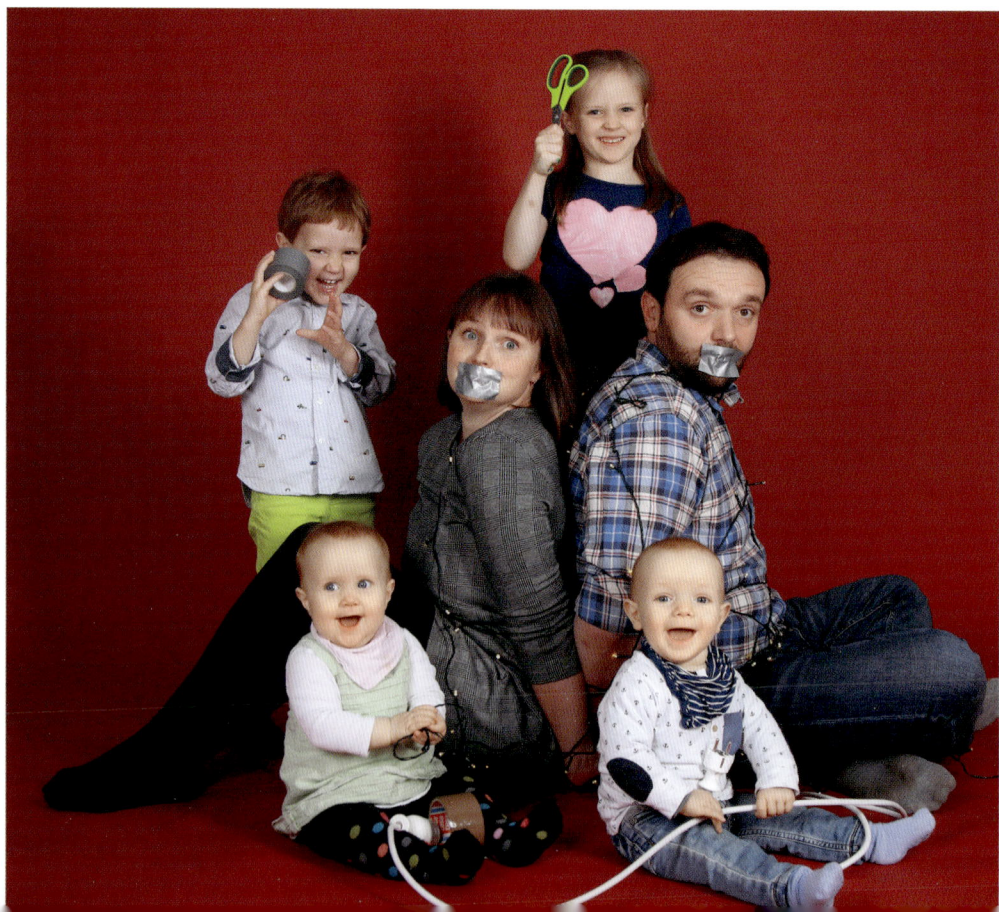

Courtesy of Sabrina Werner, smirkART Photography.

CONTENTS

FOREWORD

So it's 8 am on a Monday morning, and you get into work early to help the staff prepare for the day and to review the schedule. All good so far. Then you see at 10 am you have a new patient who is 2 years old, the child of a great patient of yours. You digest this and then start to sweat and get a bit stressed. You are not great with children, and the back door is blocked—you cannot escape! You would love to have a drink, but that is an after-work thing. You take a deep breath and call in your head assistant to help you with prep. She is amazing, as is the rest of the staff, because you trained her. Your procedures are all set up, so now what?

The child comes in and is a bit nervous, as are you. Well, fortunately you read this book and so did your staff, and you are ready to go ahead with the appointment. You smile and bend down to greet the child and hand him a sticker and ask for a hi-five. You get one in return and you now calm down—you've got this, and you will be great! Now you can take the time to enjoy the whole experience.

Working with children should not be an ordeal but a fun, rewarding experience for you and your team. Play kid music, make a balloon, and be silly like you are with your own kids. Remember that sometimes it is a slow process and you may need one or two appointments to get things done. That is fine. Also, remember that if you are good with this little one, your favorite patient will now be an even better referrer and will extol your virtues as the best dentist in town. Oftentimes, too, parents will test the waters of your office with their children, and if they do well you now have two parents as patients for life. It's helpful to appoint someone in your office to be the children coordinator. This person's job is to be the direct point of contact and help the parents and the child to have a great time and prepare them for their visit. This is the person who calms you and the patient down and is the one in charge of the fun!

This book will help prepare you for all the potential challenges and energize you for all the fun of pediatric dentistry. Remember: You would rather have a child make some noise and have no decay than have a mouth full of decay that could have been avoided. Read the book, and it's that easy. With every child you can handle, there are parents who will become your raving fans. Ulrike Uhlmann is a dear friend and colleague, and her pediatric skills and knowledge are beyond reproach. She has spent many hours creating this book to help inspire you, reward you, and help you have some fun at the same time. Take your time reading it, and make notes or highlight it when and where you can. Let your staff read this as well, as this is a great resource for them. I had a staff meeting in my practice to review it, and the response was a unanimous GREAT!

Lee Weinstein, DMD, FASDC
Pediatric Dentist and Consultant
Scottsdale, Arizona

PREFACE

I was more or less pushed into pediatric dentistry in 2010, shortly after starting to work as a general dentist. The early stages were fraught with a succession of small challenges. Of course we had learned how a pulpotomy works in our studies, but hardly any of us really had the opportunity to treat young patients ourselves.

A lot of questions do not come to light until the little kid is sitting there right in front of you. As an inexperienced dental practitioner, you constantly face situations that take you well outside your comfort zone. Children, in particular, have a keen sense of the person facing them, and you very quickly notice as a practitioner that the more confidently and purposefully you conduct yourself, the more likely you are to be successful. Back then, I benefited first and foremost from colleagues who shared their many years of experience through observation sessions and continuing education.

This book is intended as an introduction to one of the most fulfilling areas of activity in dentistry. It cannot and should not replace continuing professional development but aims to offer insight into this highly varied field. I hope I have managed to bring together fundamental knowledge that will make it easier for people taking their first steps into the field of pediatric dentistry. The structure of the book is based chronologically on a treatment session. The outcome of any treatment stands or falls by proper communication, and parents HAVE to be educated as to their vital role on the team. Examination and diagnosis then take place, followed by various treatments.

Child patients are something of a *bête noire* for many colleagues, whether they are recently qualified or have had many years on the job. Recent years have seen more focus shift to our youngest patients, with the American Academy of Pediatric Dentistry recommending a "dental home" by the time a child reaches their first birthday (see page 2). This group of patients, which is new to some dentists, raises a few questions: How do you examine a 6-month-old baby? What issues do you address with the parents? What's the appropriate fluoride prophylaxis? From what age is it reasonable to take radiographs? How do I deal with difficult children? The parents also bombard the practitioner with a host of questions—from when teeth will erupt to teething pains and advice on pacifiers to tips and tricks for daily oral hygiene in the different age groups.

Pediatric dentistry brings together a wide variety of topics encompassing all facets of dentistry, orthodontics, nutritional sciences, and, last but not least, psychology. It involves opportunity, challenge, and responsibility all at the same time. We as clinicians must ensure that even our tiniest patients get the ideal start to enable them to live with the healthiest possible oral cavity. The special challenge, of course, is not just children's compliance but primarily the fact that children can't be the ones responsible for their (oral) health. It is therefore our task to educate and motivate parents and guardians and make them our allies. A good relationship with the parents not only guarantees long-term loyalty from patients beyond their childhood years, but it is also absolutely crucial to children's good oral health. It is only when dentists manage to treat young patients properly and educate their parents that they will succeed in making a long-term contribution to children's oral health. This book therefore offers professional and practical tips on communicating with parents and sets out to illustrate the responsibility involved in treating children. Above all, it aims to garner enthusiasm in readers for this diverse field of dentistry.

Acknowledgments

Many people have played a part in the creation of this book. A big heartfelt thank you must go to Dr Lee Weinstein. He has sacrificed many hours in order to adapt the content to American guidelines and recommendations. Besides that, he contributed so many thoughts and ideas. I appreciate his work on this book very much because he is such an experienced pediatric dentist. His compassion is absolutely inspiring. Also a big thank you to Leah Huffman, Samantha Smith, and Sarah Minor, who did not become tired in view of my comments and suggestions. Thank you for putting this together. I would also like to thank Sue Holmes, who did flawless work translating the book while keeping the narrative character. Huge thanks to Anita Hattenbach and Dr Viola Lewandowski for the editing of the German version, for constantly being accessible, and for always lending a sympathetic ear to questions or ideas.

My thanks also go to those colleagues who provided numerous images from their daily practice and were thus an immense support in the production of this book. These include Dr Gabriele Viergutz (Dresden), who contributed not only several illustrations but also some important suggestions, as well as Dr Richard Steffen (Zurich), who kindly supplied photographic material from his online atlas without hesitation. My thanks also to Dr Jorge Casián Adem (Poza Rica de Hidalgo), whose high-quality photographs provided excellent documentary records. In addition, heartfelt thanks to Dr Nicola Meissner (Salzburg) for her series of photographs and her contribution. Thank you to Prof Dr Katrin Bekes (Vienna), Claudia Lippold (Halle), Dr Juliane von Hoyningen-Huene (Berlin), dental technician Peter Schaller (Munich), Dr Bobby Ghaheri (Oregon), Dr Matthias Nitsche (Leipzig), and Prof Dr Roswitha Heinrich-Weltzien (Jena) for their photographs. An enormous thank you to Sabine Fuhlbrück (Leipzig) for providing illustrations and for her tireless work on myofunctional therapy. I also owe thanks to Dr Silvia Träupmann (Leipzig) who, with her passion for pediatric dentistry and her experience, was always ready to listen to young colleagues and willingly shared her knowledge. Thank you to Manuela Richter, a highly experienced dental assistant in pediatric dentistry, who guided and supported me so much in my first cautious steps in the field. Warmest thanks to Birgit Wolff for motivating words whenever they were needed.

During the development of this book I was in contact with many inspiring colleagues, and, as a result, I was able to expand my horizons constantly and learn a lot—for which I am extremely grateful.

Last but not least, thank you to my husband who supported this project from the outset, who motivates me continually, and lightens the burden for me time and time again. Without him this book and many other accomplishments would never have been possible. Thank you.

RESOURCES

Because this book was originally published in German, much of the literature cited comes from German sources. Therefore, included below is a list of helpful resources in English for navigating the waters of pediatric dentistry.

American Academy of Pediatric Dentistry: www.aapd.org

The AAPD has many resources available on its website from scientific research on specific topics to medical history forms that can be downloaded and adapted for clinical use.

ADA MouthHealthy: www.mouthhealthy.org

This website sponsored by the American Dental Association offers practical information and resources for clinicians and parents, including free posters and activity sheets. Tips for healthy habits and a baby eruption teething chart are available at www.mouthhealthy.org/en/babies-and-kids/healthy-habits.

FDI World Dental Federation: www.fdiworlddental.org

The FDI World Dental Federation represents more than a million dentists worldwide and develops health policy and continuing education programs to promote global oral health.

American Academy of Pediatrics: www.aap.org

Dedicated to the health of all children, the AAP is a great source for new policies and guidelines for pediatric care.

US Department of Health and Human Services: www.hhs.gov

While each state has its own health and human services department, this federal branch is a good resource for information regarding social services, child or domestic abuse, and mental health.

US National Library of Medicine: www.nlm.nih.gov

Under the umbrella of the US Department of Health and Human Services, the US National Library of Medicine includes MedlinePlus, ClinicalTrials.gov, and PubMed, among other databases, all of which provide access to the latest research in all fields of medicine.

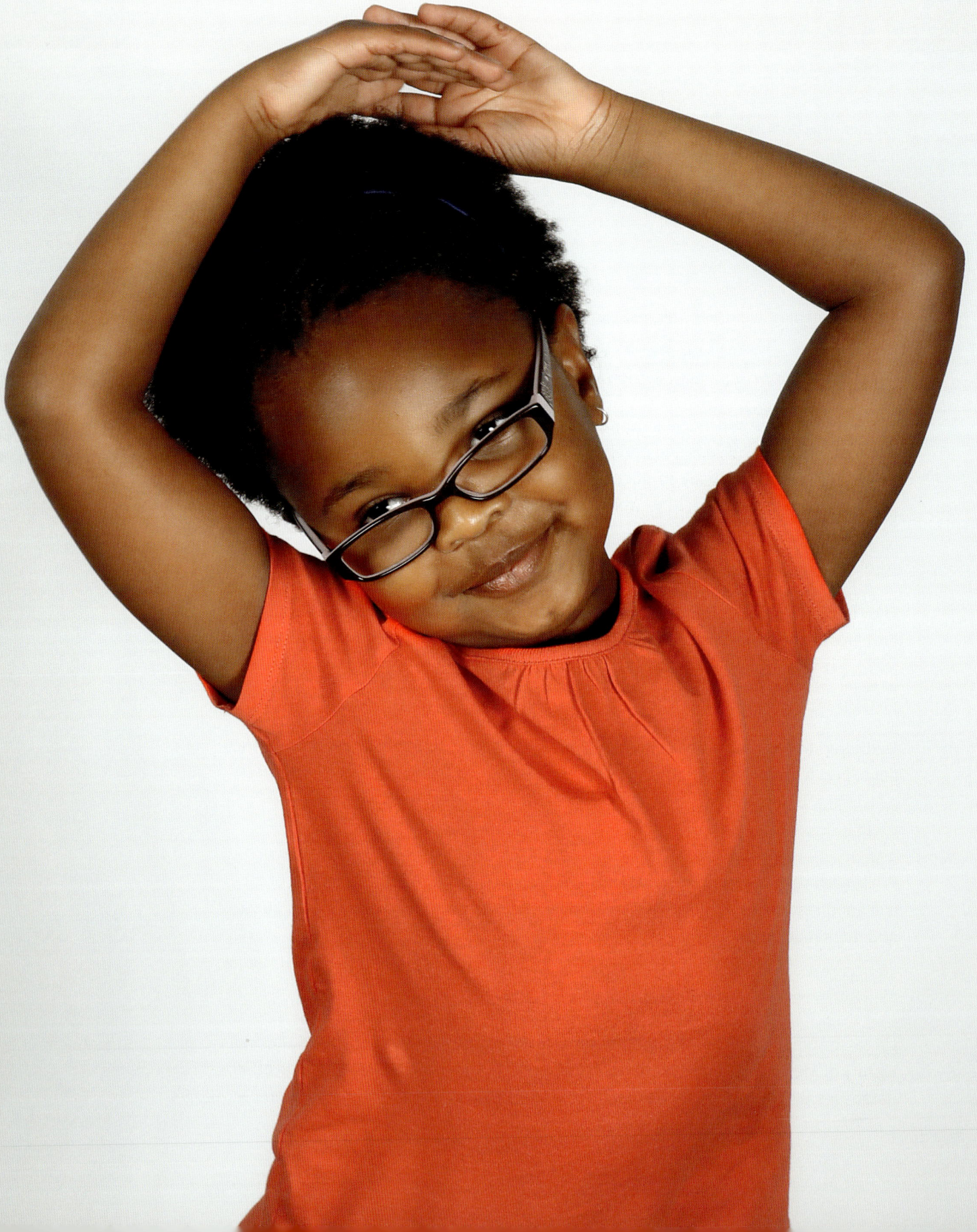

1

INTRODUCTION AND BASICS

No matter the age, children can be at times challenging, enriching, a reason to smile, as well as the cause of the odd bead of sweat on a dentist's brow! In dental prophylaxis and treatment, it is essential to adapt to these young patients in order to achieve the best treatment outcomes, guarantee long-term patient loyalty, and, perhaps most importantly, ensure that these patients of tomorrow do not grow up anxious under our care. According to estimates, around two-thirds of anxious adult patients link their anxiety to a traumatic experience with a dentist in their childhood.[1]

In dental school, we are faced with a lot of theory, but there is virtually no discussion of the practical aspects of treating children. Because it is sometimes impossible to reconcile theory and practice without a degree of compromise, especially in pediatric dentistry, the treatment of young patients often poses a challenge in everyday practice. In many practices, seasoned dentists prefer that treatment of children is performed by the newest hire just out of dental school or with the most junior status; however, they often do not have the necessary communication skills to improve or maintain compliance from young patients. Nonetheless, provided the diagnostic steps run smoothly and none or only minor findings become apparent, no one involved has to leave their comfort zone. But what if measures become necessary that demand more from the patient and practitioner than their individual comfort zones will allow?

Children are incredibly receptive and attuned to the people interacting with them. Uncertainties are easily transmitted to young patients, which commonly results in stress and refusal. Specialized pediatric dentists are often called in too late and then laboriously have to regain the child's trust. But it can be different! With a few tricks in organization, communication, and treatment; proper diagnostic testing; and realistic recognition of one's own capabilities and limitations, treatment of children can become established as a successful element of a practice concept.

> "Only those who attempt the absurd can achieve the impossible."
>
> ALBERT EINSTEIN

The concept of a family dental practice yields benefits for all those involved: Parents can combine their preventive care appointments with their children's to save time, while dentists can gain a whole new patient base and duplicate their range of treatments and that of their team. Treating children also provides dentists with more variety in everyday work, opens up new prospects, and creates trust. Parents who know their children are in good hands with a dentist will be happy to become or remain patients themselves.

The great challenge in pediatric dentistry is determining which treatment approach and technique is most appropriate for each individual patient. Not every young patient is suitable for classic filling therapy, and the wait-and-see approach after fluoride application is not appropriate for many children. However, it should still be our main goal to provide even our youngest patients with optimal, state-of-the-art treatment.

In addition, we must not forget that pediatric dentistry in particular is much more than just drill and fill. Our actual core task and daily challenge is prophylaxis and the prevention of caries. Unlike adult patients, children are not able to take responsibility for their own oral health. There is no reason for caries to develop in primary teeth, and yet, on a daily basis, we see that the reality is quite different. This is why we need to partner with parents and make them understand that they are the key to their children's oral health. Sometimes this can be a considerable challenge.

The objective of the first dental examination is to fully inform parents about the relevant topics (fluoride, oral hygiene, diet, drinking), dispel any fears (eg, premature or delayed eruption of teeth, grinding teeth, teething troubles), and detect or prevent early childhood caries (ECC). This visit also serves to familiarize children with dental treatment in a positive way so that they are less anxious for future visits that may be required for trauma or caries. Most importantly, the purpose of these early visits is to establish a "dental home" for the child and their parents.

DENTAL HOME

The American Academy of Pediatric Dentistry (AAPD) defines a dental home as the "ongoing relationship between the dentist and the patient, inclusive of all aspects of oral health care delivered in a comprehensive, continuously accessible, coordinated, and family-centered way. The dental home should be established no later than 12 months of age to help children and their families institute a lifetime of good oral health. A dental home addresses anticipatory guidance and preventive, acute, and comprehensive oral health care and includes referral to dental specialists when appropriate" (AAPD, 2018). Our care should always be centered around the child, meaning that if we can't offer proper treatment, we refer to someone who we think can; the referral of a patient does not mean we failed doing our job but rather that we care for our patients more than for our ego. For this we will not lose any patients but gain trust and thankfulness.

This introductory chapter briefly addresses the most important anatomical, physiologic, and morphologic basics of primary teeth that have practical relevance. This chapter may also be used as a source for mineralization and eruption times as well as the multifactorial etiology of caries. The teething charts can also be copied and handed out to parents.

STRUCTURE OF PRIMARY TEETH

The structure of primary teeth differs significantly from that of permanent teeth, and this factor has a direct influence on treatment. First, a few particular features must be kept in mind during adhesive cementation of fillings because of the morphologic characteristics of primary teeth (Box 1-1). Second, caries in primary teeth invades the dentin more quickly and endodontic treatments are required far earlier than with permanent teeth because of the macromorphology of primary teeth (Fig 1-1).

The micromorphology is characterized by an aprismatic and irregular enamel structure (Fig 1-2). The proportion of organic constituents is higher than in permanent teeth, which explains poorer conditioning by the acid etch technique. The dentin structure also differs from that of permanent teeth (Fig 1-3): The mineral content is reduced, the distribution of dentinal tubules is more irregular, and the tubules are larger. This explains the faster progression of caries and the lower dentin adhesive values.[3]

BOX 1-1 Morphologic characteristics of primary teeth[2]

Macromorphology
- The enamel mantle is not thicker than 1 mm in any location.
- The pulp chamber of the primary teeth is relatively larger, and the pulp horns are relatively more exposed compared with permanent teeth.
- The occlusal surfaces of the primary teeth are narrower in comparison to permanent teeth, and their buccal and lingual facets diverge toward a strongly developed cervical or basal enamel bulge.
- Primary molars have a broader and flatter interproximal contact than permanent molars.

Micromorphology
- The enamel surface is characterized by a largely aprismatic enamel surface (layer thickness 30–100 μm).
- The enamel prisms in the cervical area increase from the dentinoenamel junction toward the occlusal surface.
- The mineral content of the primary tooth enamel is lower than in the permanent dentition.
- In primary teeth the enamel formed postnatally is far less densely mineralized than the prenatal enamel mantle.
- The structure of primary tooth dentin is different than permanent tooth dentin: The dentinal tubules are larger, the peritubular dentin is more highly developed, and the mineral content of the intertubular dentin is lower than in the permanent dentition.

Fig 1-1 Morphologic differences between primary and permanent teeth.

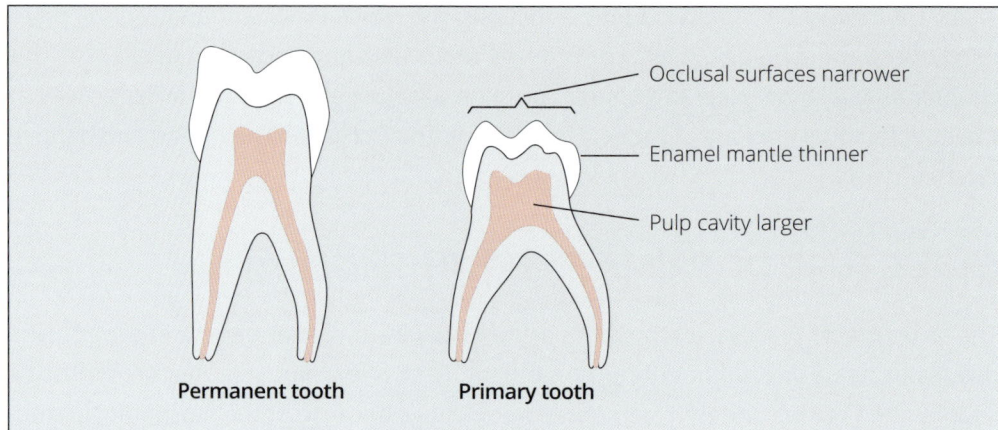

Occlusal surfaces narrower

Enamel mantle thinner

Pulp cavity larger

Permanent tooth   Primary tooth

Fig 1-2 Cross section of a primary *(a)* versus a permanent *(b)* tooth revealing enamel layer thickness. In the primary tooth, the enamel layer is very thin compared with the permanent tooth. (Photographs courtesy of Peter Schaller.)

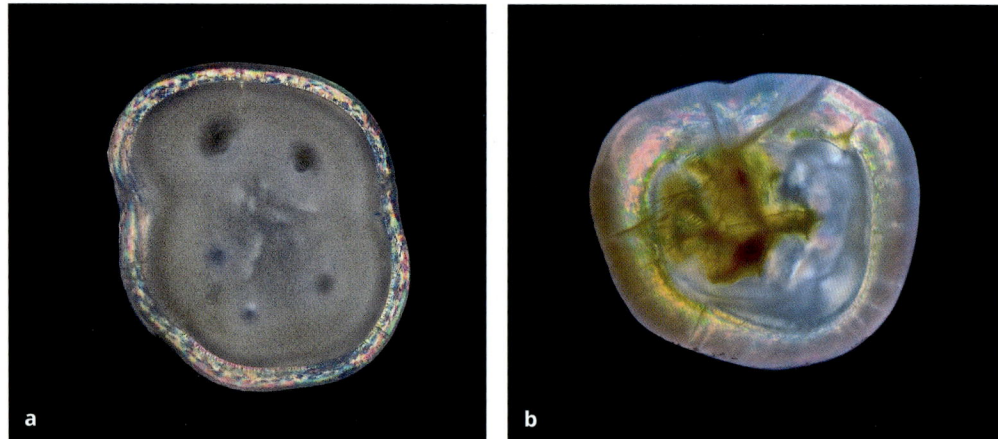

Fig 1-3 Longitudinal section of a primary *(a)* versus a permanent *(b)* tooth. The size of the pulp cavity is much larger in the primary tooth, whereas the dentin layer between the enamel and the pulp is much thicker in the permanent tooth. (Photographs courtesy of Peter Schaller.)

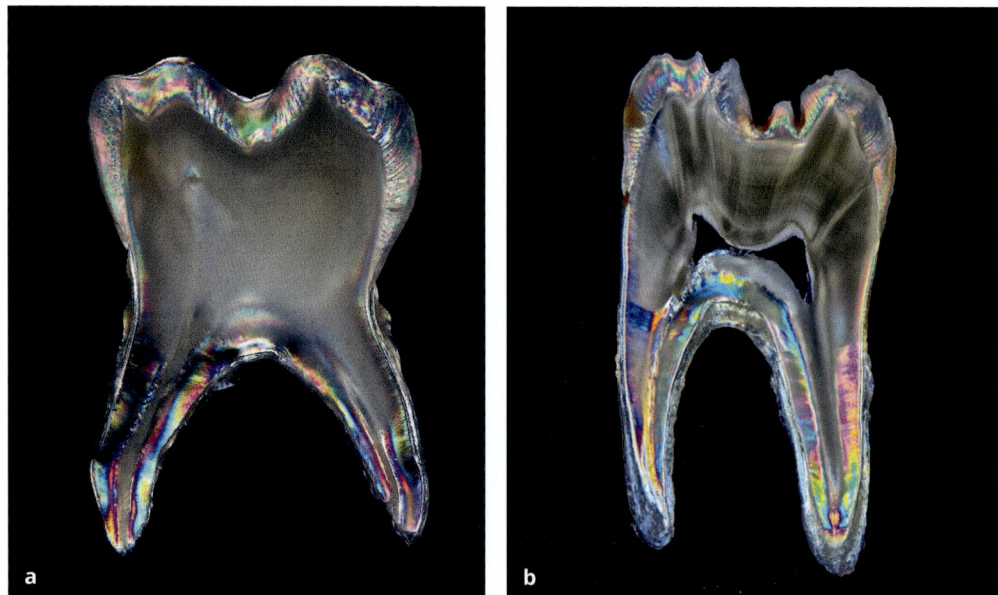

TABLE 1-1 Mineralization times of the primary teeth[4]

Tooth	Start of mineralization	End of mineralization	Root fully developed
Incisors	3–5 months in utero	4–5 months post-natal	1.5–2 years
Canines	5 months in utero	9 months postnatal	2.5–3 years
Primary first molar	5 months in utero	6 months postnatal	2–2.75 years
Primary second molar	6–7 months in utero	10–12 months postnatal	3 years

TABLE 1-2 Mineralization times of the permanent teeth[4]

Tooth	Start of mineralization	Crown fully developed	Root fully developed
Maxilla			
Central incisor	3–4 months	4–5 years	10 years
Lateral incisor	Up to 1 year	4–5 years	11 years
Canine	4–5 months	6–7 years	13–15 years
First premolar	1.5–1.75 years	5–6 years	13–15 years
Second premolar	2–2.25 years	6–7 years	12–14 years
First molar	At birth	2.5–3 years	9–10 years
Second molar	2.5–3 years	7–8 years	14–16 years
Third molar	7–9 years	12–16 years	18–25 years
Mandible			
Central incisor	3–4 months	4–5 years	9 years
Lateral incisor	3–4 months	4–5 years	10 years
Canine	4–5 months	6–7 years	12–14 years
First premolar	1.75–2 years	5–6 years	13 years
Second premolar	2.25–2.5 years	6–7 years	13–14 years
First molar	At birth	2.5–3 years	9–10 years
Second molar	2.5–3 years	7–8 years	14–15 years
Third molar	8–10 years	12–16 years	18–25 years

MINERALIZATION AND ERUPTION TIMES

To understand disorders such as hypomineralization or dental fluorosis, we need to know exactly when primary and permanent teeth are mineralized (Tables 1-1 and 1-2). Furthermore, when assessing radiographs in the mixed dentition, it can be helpful to know when the dental crowns of the permanent premolars or molars should be visible

TABLE 1-3 Eruption times of the primary and permanent teeth*

Tooth	Eruption times
Primary	
Central incisor	6–8 months
Lateral incisor	8–12 months
First molar	12–16 months
Canine	16–20 months
Second molar	20–30 months
Permanent	
First molar (6-year molar)	5–7 years
Central incisor	6–8 years
Lateral incisor	7–9 years
Canines and premolars	9–12 years
Second molar (12-year molar)	11–14 years
Third molar (wisdom tooth)	16+ years

* Relatively wide variations in these timings are possible.

so that any agenesis can be diagnosed. Table 1-3 shows the eruption times of the primary and permanent teeth. It should be noted that relatively wide variations in these timings are possible; those listed in the table should only serve as a guide.

CARIES AS A MULTIFACTORIAL DISEASE

Because caries is a multifactorial disease, it is up to the clinician to identify each patient's individual risk factors and intervene preventively and therapeutically in a targeted way. Especially in children who have no influence on their own diet and oral hygiene, it is important to identify all the etiologic factors contributing to the caries so that adjustments can be made, provided the parents are compliant and reliable, to achieve a lasting reduction of the risk of caries. Figure 1-4 represents the caries etiology model[5] according to Fejerskov and Kidd, illustrating the various key components and their interactions for the purpose of successful caries assessment.

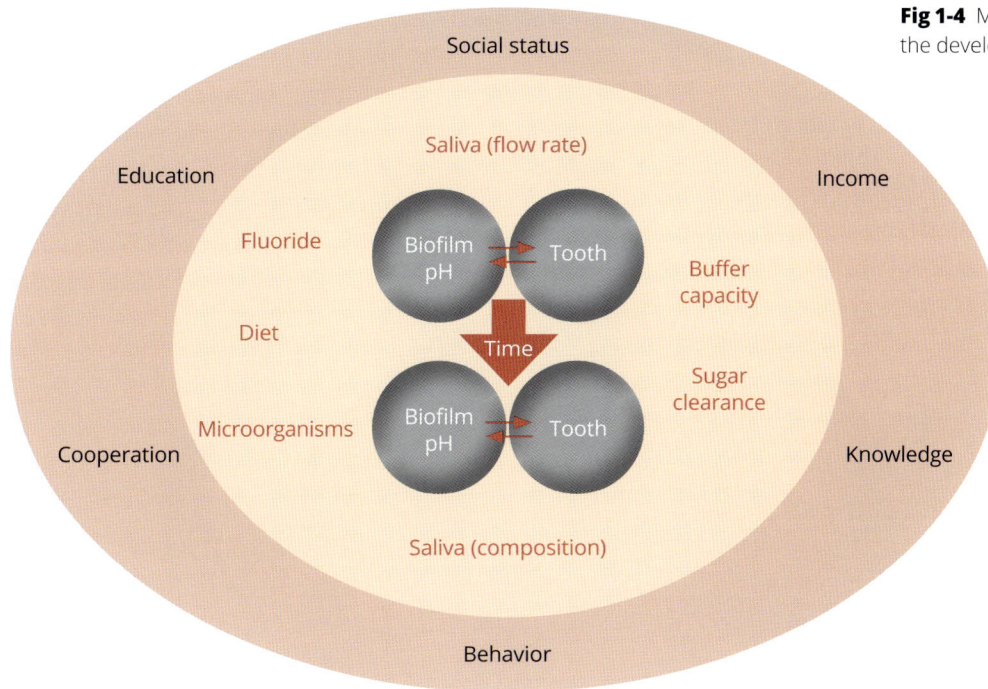

Fig 1-4 Multifactorial etiology model of the development of caries.

REFERENCES

1. Müller EM, Hasslinger Y. Sprechen Sie schon Kind?: Prophylaxe auf Augenhöe. Berlin: Quintessenz, 2016.
2. Ermler R. Diagnostik von Approximalkaries bei Milchmolaren mit Hilfe des DIAGNOdent pen. Berlin: Charité, Universitätsmedizin Berlin, 2009.
3. van Waes H, Stöckli P (eds). Kinderzahnmedizin, Farbatlanten der Zahnmedizin. Stuttgart: Thieme, 2001.
4. Mittelsdorf A. Kariesprävention mit Fluoriden – Eine Fragebogenaktion zur Fluoridverordnung in Berliner Kinderarztpraxen unter besonderer Berücksichtigung der Empfehlungen der DGZMK. Berlin: Charité, Universitätsmedizin Berlin, 2010.
5. Kühnisch J, Hickel R, Heinrich-Weltzien R. Kariesrisiko und Kariesaktivität. Quintessenz 2010;61:271–280.

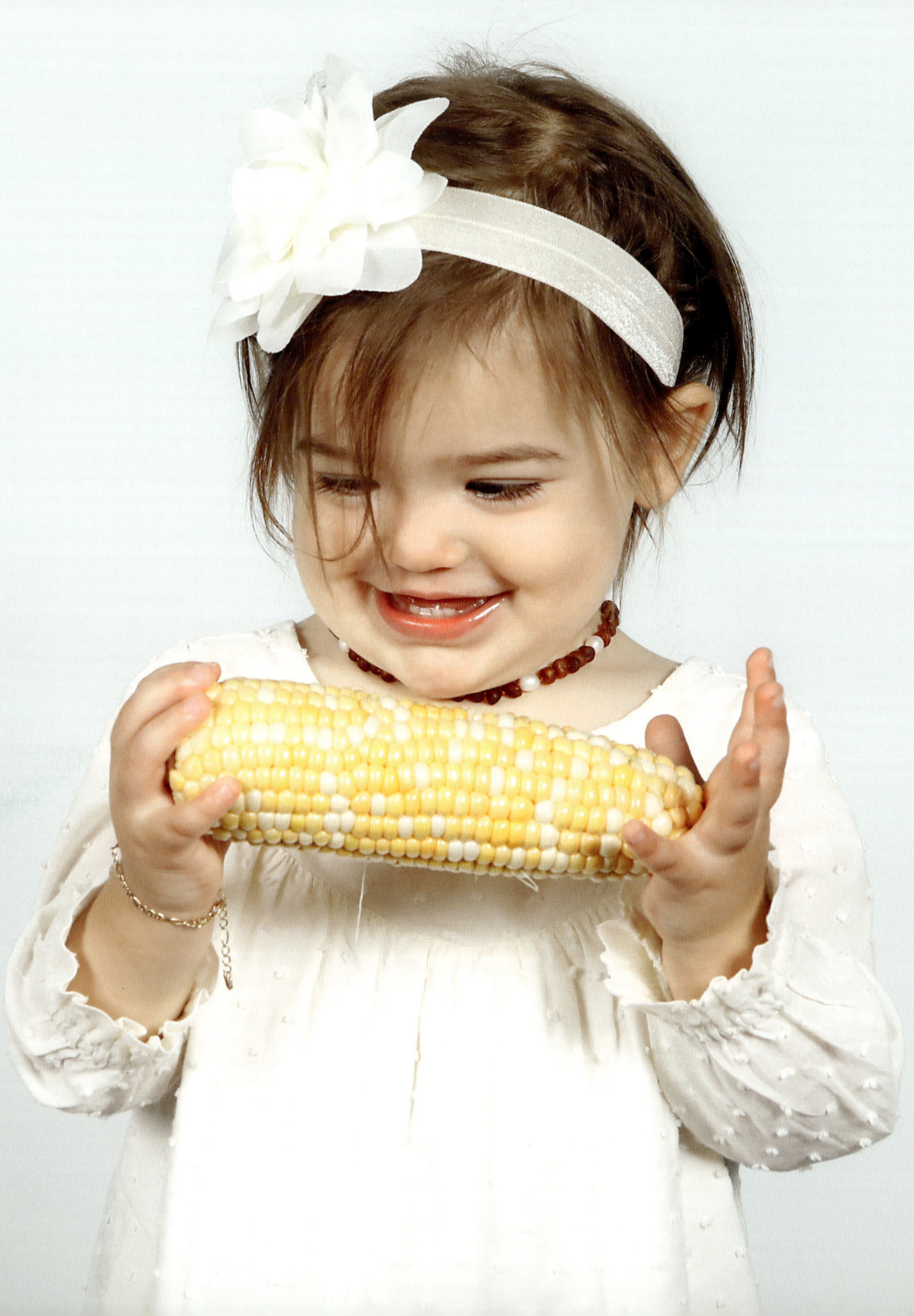

2

SUCCESSFUL COMMUNICATION WITH KIDS AND PARENTS

Communication with your pediatric patient begins not when the treatment starts but as soon as the child enters the dental practice. Communication is not merely about talking; it includes a plethora of nonverbal signals. American-Austrian psychologist Paul Watzlawick expressed this clearly when he said "You cannot not communicate." Communication consists of 55% nonverbal cues (gestures and facial expressions), 38% tone of voice, and only 7% actual content of what is said.[2] This chapter examines the different levels of communication and their importance in the dental practice. Suggestions are then given regarding how to use verbal and nonverbal language to gain, improve, or maintain compliance for different types of pediatric patients.

IMPORTANCE OF CHILD-APPROPRIATE ENVIRONMENT

Children need to be engaged to feel comfortable in any public space. General dentistry practices without a specialization in pediatric treatment can create a child-friendly environment with just a few resources. To do this, it is helpful and necessary to visualize the viewpoint of a child; they first see what is at their eye level or below it. Pictures, wall stickers, or even toys in the waiting room should be placed at a height where children can see and reach. A coloring table, some well-chosen books, and a set of building blocks are sufficient to create an engaging environment for children. If space is a concern, there are also some brilliant space-saving play alternatives, such as wall-mounted drawing boards, magnetic boards, jigsaw puzzles, or games. Wooden toys are often a more robust and durable choice. In the interests of other patients and the practice team, toys that emit sounds are inadvisable. When selecting toys for a common space, consider the cleansability; toys that are hard to sanitize may prove poor choices during flu season. In

"The use of humor in pediatric dentistry is highly recommended. It may be used to facilitate communications with patients and parents, alleviate patient anxiety, and assist the dentist in coping with stress associated with the practice of dentistry."

MOSTOFSKY AND FORTUNE[1]

9

addition, wall decals are a useful and variable design feature for the waiting room or a treatment room because they are easy to remove without leaving a mark.

Not every dentist has the facility to mount a monitor above the treatment chair; as a more convenient alternative, a photo or painting on the ceiling will not only fascinate young children but will also help to distract older, anxious patients. Finally, the reception counter often seems enormous to children, so a small stool can make it a little more manageable for curious children to sneak a peek. Air freshener spray should be kept on hand as well to eliminate the typical smells of the dental practice, which can unsettle or frighten some children.

NONVERBAL COMMUNICATION, INDIVIDUAL PERSONAL SPACE, AND PROXIMITY

"You cannot not communicate."

PAUL WATZLAWICK

Children are particularly sensitive to nonverbal signals communicated by body language, such as gestures and facial expressions.[3] Because nonverbal communication is unconsciously controlled by our thoughts, it is important to always have a positive attitude that enables us to communicate authentically and empathetically—especially in the company of children with behavioral problems. Children have a very keen sense of how well physical and verbal signals match each other—if they do not, the intended message will be misunderstood. Thus, the treatment of a child with behavioral issues may fail from the outset if the dentist exhibits antipathy but tries to cover it up. Children are highly sensitive to discrepancies between what is said and what is felt.[4]

One of the greatest challenges in the practice of pediatric dentistry is controlling the often-unconscious nonverbal signals we send out so that the young patient gets a positive impression. Especially when beginning with pediatric treatment, self-reflection and analysis of these nonverbal (and verbal) signals is key. Important positive signals include an open smile, a calm manner, and nonjerky movements. Equally important is a respect for the individual child's personal space—the personal space that they need to feel safe and secure. If people invade our personal space against our will, it can result in rejection, aggression, and anxiety, so we should not expect children to react any differently. While we generally think of any violation of this space in terms of physical proximity, personal space can also be breached nonverbally with a look or a gesture.[3] Note that anxious children generally require a larger personal space than outgoing children do.

Therefore, it is important for dentists and dental assistants to read, interpret, and respect a child's signals when interacting with them. At the same time, however, this personal space needs to be shrunk enough to make dental treatment possible. This is often where the real challenge lies. It calls for patience, a slow approach, acceptance, positive nonverbal signals, rituals (eg, similar sequence when greeting patients or going about the treatment), and sometimes even the patient's stuffed animals or toys to act as neutral mediators. Once comfortable, children will allow the dentist to encroach on their personal space, and a neutral approach can often be adopted. Stuffed animals can also be a great advantage during treatment: They can be used to demonstrate to the child what the dentist is going to do, thereby allaying the child's fears, or they can reflect the child's behavior and thus be used to alter that behavior.[3] For example, the dentist can use a hand puppet to mimic a child's resistance (eg, refusing to open their mouth) and then convince the puppet to let itself be examined, rewarding it with praise and maybe even a small prize. This can influence the child's behavior and often positively change their attitude. It is not uncommon to see young patients reflect the behavior of the stuffed animal (eg, by opening their mouth).

As mentioned initially, these aspects do not only have a bearing when the child sits down in the dentist's chair but as soon as the child enters the practice. A friendly smile from the dental assistant at reception and greeting the young patient by name while respecting the patient's personal space will pave the way for a successful start. When greeting or calling a child from the waiting room, it is important to get down to the child's eye level. Anything else has an intimidating and threatening effect. On first contact in the waiting room, the ideal distance to maintain from the patient is about 1 m (3 ft). The child should be greeted before his or her parents. Personal information that can be obtained from the case history (eg, the name of the stuffed animal or the child's favorite color) makes it easier to establish contact and create trust. In doing so, it is important to be authentic and empathetic. If it becomes clear that the child is very anxious or agitated, do not tell them that what they are feeling is not necessary. Telling a child that "there's no reason to be nervous" is well intentioned but will not reassure a child. On the contrary, it creates additional insecurity because children learn that the feelings they are experiencing are wrong. It is better to show empathy by saying, "I can see you're pretty nervous. I can understand that. I'll explain everything to you exactly. That'll help you feel comfortable."

To maintain this first connection, once established, it is important for the young patient to be accompanied into the treatment room. This can be used as an opportunity to explain what things you might notice along the way (sounds, smells, or images), or the dentist can give an idea of what is going to happen in the treatment room.[5] If the dental assistant brings the child into the treatment room, he or she should introduce the dentist and explain to the child what will happen next.

During the treatment, it is an important part of nonverbal communication for dentists or dental assistants to reassure the child with appropriate touch as soon as they have a hand free. An assistant's hand on the shoulder, tummy, or head (especially the temples), for instance, conveys a feeling of care and protection and may set the child more at ease.[6] At the same time, various acupressure points can be massaged during the treatment (see chapter 7). By contrast, stroking is often counterproductive because it may increase a child's awareness of being touched. Be aware of this nonverbal communication, and if it is clear that the child is uncomfortable with any of this touching, stop it at once.

VERBAL COMMUNICATION: THE RIGHT CHOICE OF WORDS

Even though children are often preconditioned by their family ("If you don't clean your teeth properly, you'll have to go to the dentist and he'll drill them"), we as dentists are responsible for shaping children's positive experiences with our profession. Generally speaking, voice control is needed when dealing with young patients: different phases of treatment can be accompanied by different tones of voice and/or levels of loudness. For example, while the treatment is going on, the dentist should talk in a monotone voice that is not too loud. If a child tries to touch the syringe, for instance, he or she can be stopped in a friendly way but with a louder voice. If the child is constantly crying or whimpering, a quiet whispering voice can be used, and the child's curiosity about what is being said may silence the crying.[7]

Child-appropriate language is another foundation of successful pediatric treatment. This means using simple, short sentences without any complicated or foreign words. Before the age of 5 years, children cannot grasp abstract expressions of time (afterward, then, later, etc), which can easily be a cause of frustration. In addition, it can be very helpful for the dentist to be reasonably familiar with the latest children's movies or TV series. This can be a way of gaining the young patient's trust. The dental practitioner must be sensitive and reflect on his or her choice of words, especially when explaining equipment or treatment steps. If a toddler has only ever heard of a drill from daddy's tool box, it is understandably frightening if the word is used in connection with their own mouth. (Table 2-1 offers suggestions for child-appropriate terms for dental instruments.) Children have a fertile imagination, which the dentist can readily tap into. In the beginning it may involve some effort to open yourself up to this world of imagination and create a story to explain the treatment and put the child's mind at ease. Stories can help to distract young patients and make them far more relaxed during a dental treatment.

Inappropriate use of "okay" can pose another problem. We are often accustomed to ending a sentence with this word, but children frequently understand it as a question. It can become a bit of a challenge if a sentence such as "I'm now going to rinse your tooth clean, okay," is answered by the child with a definite "no."[5] Generally questions by the dentist should be used very specifically. Before children reach preschool age, it is helpful to ask questions like, "What games do you like playing?" in order to build up a conversation. Communication can be established because children are then obliged to answer with a sentence and not just "yes" or "no."[3] Once children have reached preschool age, alternative questions can be employed that invite the child to make pseudodecisions, like "Do you want to climb up onto the chair by yourself, or do you want mom or dad to get up first and you can sit on their lap?" However, the dentist should make sure only to offer alternatives that are equally conducive to the ongoing treatment process.

Praise and reward are important elements when working with children. Young patients should be praised for a particular reason. There is no point in rewarding a child with something if the child has been thoroughly uncooperative; this tells these patients that their behavior was acceptable. It is more helpful to say exactly what you were pleased about and praise the patient for that. For example: "Today you came with us into the treatment room really nicely and you let me have a look at your front teeth. That was very good, so I'm going to give you a little prize. Next time I'd like you to open your mouth really wide so I can count all your teeth." This can give the child an idea and an expectation about the next treatment.[5] Praise during treatment is also an important motivating tool.

TABLE 2-1 Suggestions for correct choice of words

Instrument	Child-appropriate term(s)
Lamp	Sun
Probe	Tooth feeler; tooth counter
Suction	Magic wand that carries away spit; snorkel; drinking straw; vacuum
Red contra-angle or turbine (water)	Shower; water sprayer
Blue contra-angle	Tickle bee
Excavator	Little spoon
Syringe	Sleeping water; sleeping medicine
Etching gel	Smurf cream; tooth shampoo
Curing lamp	Magic lantern; light saber
Composite or other filling materials	Magic cream
Cotton wool rolls	Pillows for your tooth
Rubber dam	Raincoat for your tooth
Matrix	Gold or silver medals for your tooth (depending on the color of the matrix)
Wooden wedge	Garden fence
Forceps	Mini-crane
Caries, tooth decay	Sugar bugs
Steel crown	Knight's or princess's tooth
Treatment chair	Kiddie throne; lounger; up-and-down chair; magic chair
Air blower	Hairdryer or air pistol
Water spout	Waterfall

Phrases like "You're opening your mouth so well" and "You're sitting so nicely" can really go a long way to making the child feel more comfortable and good about themselves.

At the end of treatment, the wrong behavior by parents or accompanying persons can also be problematic. Empathy is important, but exaggerated expressions of sympathy reinforce the child's impression that the dental treatment was something traumatic, which in future will cause the child to be afraid.[5] To avoid such situations, it can be helpful before dental treatments to issue parents with a brief guide on what to do (Fig 2-1). In general it is important to end a treatment session with positive feedback and a little reward for the child, for example, a sticker or other prize.

Dear Parent,

A visit to the dentist is an exciting new experience for your child. In order to ensure that it's a positive experience, we would like to give you a few tips on how you can help us and your child. Even if some of this advice might seem unusual, you can be sure that this approach has been effective in a lot of treatments of children.

A child is not a little adult!

Before the treatment
Your child should be rested and relaxed when attending the appointment. Arouse your child's curiosity about the visit to the dentist beforehand and avoid transferring any fears you may have to your child. We will introduce your child to any treatment in a playful way. It will be like magic, and we might even "count" the teeth of your child's favorite stuffed animal.

Communication
Please avoid well-intended sentences such as "You don't need to be frightened" or "It won't hurt at all." These phrases make your child think something might happen that *will* hurt or that he or she *ought* to be frightened. Sentences like "You see, that wasn't so bad" at the end of the treatment are unhelpful as well. We only use positive, child-appropriate words for our instruments and all treatment steps, so at home please try to avoid words like "drill," "syringe," or "pull out." Even if your child says, "That's a syringe" when with us, we follow the same practice and will answer, "No, it's a sleeping medicine for your tooth."

During the treatment
Please stay in the background during the treatment, even if it is difficult for you. This makes it easier for us to establish contact and communicate with your child.

After the treatment
Do not promise your child any presents as a reward. This sort of thing places your child under too much pressure during the treatment and makes it difficult for us to work. Your child will get praise from us during and after the treatment and, of course, can choose a little prize afterward.

If things don't go so well...
There is a possibility that a treatment might not go quite so well, especially if your child has had negative experiences in the past or if they are particularly anxious. Please don't scold your child about this. We will still try to find a positive end to the treatment, and together we will discuss a strategy for further action.

We hope your child—and you as parents—will feel perfectly comfortable with us!

Thank you!
Your practice team

Fig 2-1 Example letter giving parents advice on what to do to improve their child's experience at the dentist.

TELL-SHOW-DO METHOD

The "tell-show-do" method combines the most important levels of communication (*tell* = verbal, *show* = nonverbal) and also addresses another sensory level: feeling. This technique is therefore ideal for explaining treatment steps to children. During the execution part of the method (*do*), the sensations that are to be expected should therefore be mimicked. For instance, the pressure from the rubber dam clamp or the extracting forceps can be imitated by pressing the hand on the child's shoulder. With very nervous children, it may be advisable to demonstrate all the actions first on yourself or on a hand puppet. In an expansion of the method (tell-show-ask-do), the dental practitioner obtains the child's consent before performing the actions and only continues once the child has signaled his or her agreement.[3]

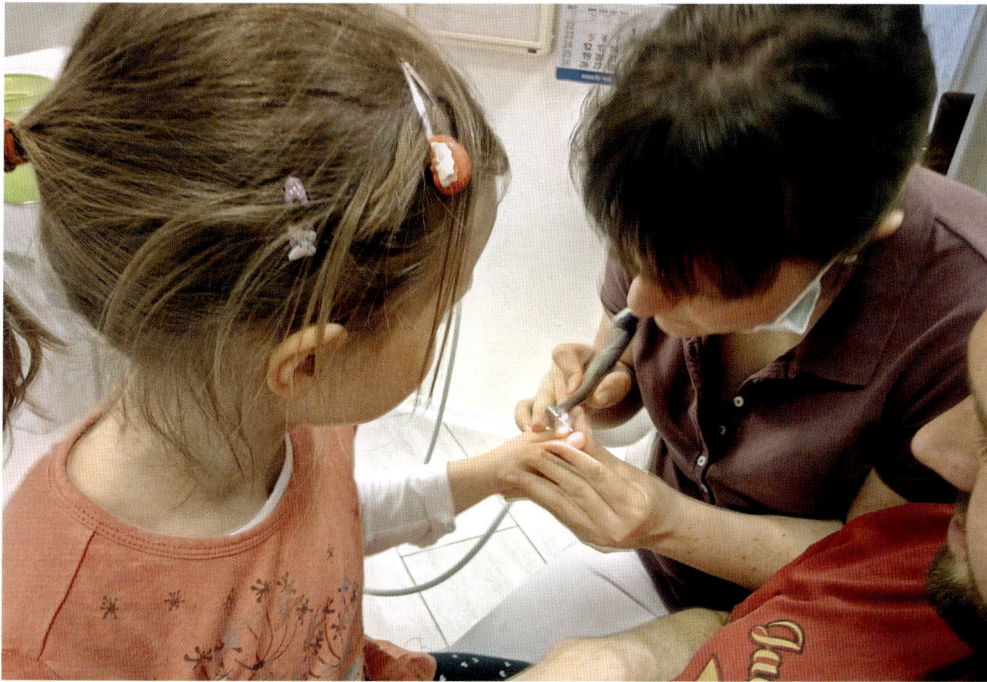

Fig 2-2 Tell-show-do method on a 4-year-old patient. A round bur is being demonstrated on the little girl's fingernail. You can use the bur to "paint" a sun on the child's nail, for example, then repeat the same thing on the tooth.

It is important to make sure you only explain or demonstrate the different treatment steps immediately before carrying them out (Fig 2-2). Because children have a short attention span, there is no point in explaining all the steps just at the beginning.

BASIC RULES FOR COMMUNICATION WITH CHILDREN IN THE DENTAL PRACTICE
Nonverbal: Be authentic, focus on the child, ensure there is a congruence between what the dentist feels and says, smile genuinely, use smooth movements, respect personal space, be patient, take the child seriously, let the child finish speaking, establish contact by appropriate touch during treatment (ie, touching the shoulder or the temples), communicate at eye level, and perform ritualized actions.
Verbal: Control your voice, show (not exaggerated) empathy, avoid denials or negative sentences, do not use unfamiliar foreign words, avoid irony/sarcasm, use descriptive language, talk in a low and calm tone of voice, keep sentences short and simple, be careful about questions ending with "okay," allow for patient involvement in noncritical decisions (ie, getting in chair alone or with parent), choose positive words, and offer praise during and after treatment.
Other: Hypnosis, behavior management, and acupressure are auxiliary methods that can be used.[6]

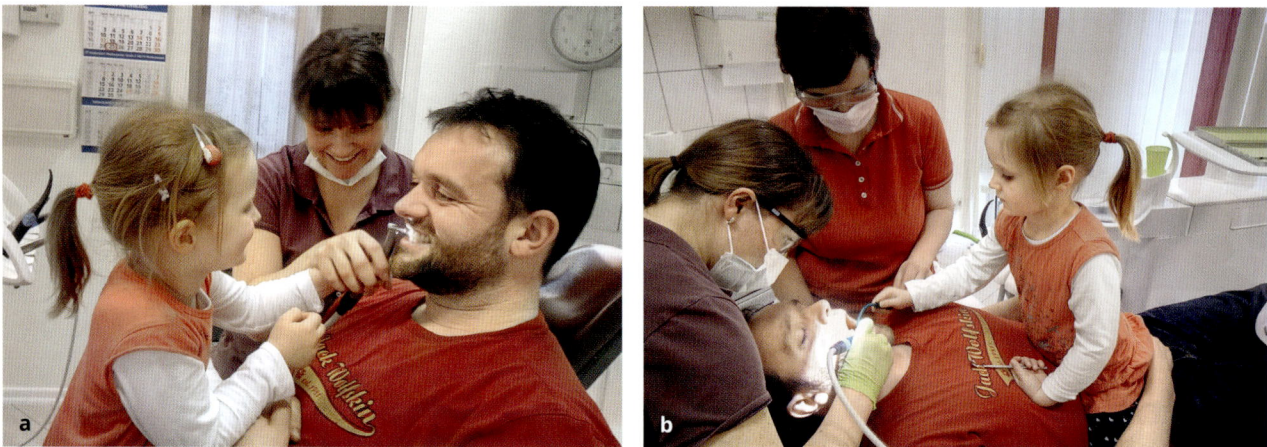

Fig 2-3 *(a)* Demonstrating a brush on daddy. *(b)* This young patient was able to use the suction and "examine" daddy's teeth with a little mirror.

DIFFERENT TYPES OF PEDIATRIC PATIENTS AND PARENTS

Constant criers

This type of young patient will cry constantly even without any discernible reason. It can help to talk extra quietly to these children. This often arouses their curiosity and they quiet down so that they can actually understand what is being said. Dentists who are comfortable singing can utilize the element of surprise and start singing a children's song a little louder than the child's crying. Many children will then stop in surprise. Then you can continue singing quietly and start/continue the examination.

Extremely shy patients

Extremely shy patients will hide under a chair or behind a person they trust (ie, a parent) while still in the waiting room. These children need a lot of time and space to settle into the new situation. It is important to accept the personal space that the individual child needs and not crowd the patient. It can help to ignore the child completely and solely address the parent, who is examined by the tell-show-do method. While the parent is being examined, all the findings are communicated to the dental assistant in a child-appropriate way ("I've counted eight of mommy's teeth and they are lovely and sparkling"), and cooperative behavior is praised and rewarded in a way that is obvious to the child. These patients will often lose some of their shyness as their parents are being examined and take a curious look into their parent's mouth or want to hold the mirror (Fig 2-3). Occasionally the prize at the end of examination will tempt them and will boost cooperation.

It is important not to put pressure on this type of patient and expect too much of them. Investing a little more time at the outset will pay off later. Sometimes two appointments may be necessary to examine these children.

> **CAUTION**
>
> If the parents are anxious patients themselves, it is not advisable to examine the parents by way of example. Overstressing anxious and nervous parents is not productive and tends to create mistrust in the child.

Know-it-alls

These young patients think they know everything about all the treatment steps and like to share their knowledge with the dentist. It can be difficult to sell a syringe to these children as "sleeping medicine." Sentences such as "I know that's a syringe and not 'sleeping medicine'" can easily put the dentist and dental assistant off their stride. It is helpful to reflect the children's behavior and show off with a foreign word, for instance, saying, "You're absolutely right, it's not 'sleeping medicine' but anesthesia." This rebuttal can elicit a suitable reaction from the young patient. The child learns something he or she did not know before, and the dentist remains master of the situation.

Overly spoiled children

The particularly spoiled child is one of the most difficult patients in daily practice. They often confront the dentist petulantly and are defended in their behavior by their parents. Without actually being afraid of the upcoming treatment, they refuse to cooperate. In these cases, dentists can use voice control to their advantage, speaking calmly and more quietly if it is working well. If the child does not cooperate, the dentist speaks more loudly in a more assertive tone of voice. Furthermore, a timed ultimatum can be set during which the child has to go back and sit in the waiting room. If the child entirely refuses to cooperate, a new appointment is made in 2 to 3 weeks.[8] Sometimes it may be more advisable to separate the child from the parents for the examination or the treatment.

These children are often raised in anti-authoritarian households with few boundaries and are simply transferring this behavior to the dental practice. The result is a constant testing and challenging, for instance, pressing the buttons on the treatment unit without asking or being disrespectful toward the dentist or practice personnel ("You're dumb and no way am I going to let you look in my mouth!"). It is important to communicate the rules clearly to these children: "Please listen to me. This is my practice and in here we work by my rules. I'd like you to be nice to me and everyone working here—just as nice as you expect me to be. I cannot keep your teeth healthy if you disrespect me and my helpers and mess with all of my instruments." These children generally accept these boundaries and usually can be treated without any more difficulty.

Helicopter parents

"Helicopter parents" can make life difficult for you as the dentist, especially if you are fairly young. They are excessively protective of their children, constantly interfering verbally in the treatment, and questioning everything first. This can prevent the dentist from establishing a connection with the child because he or she is continually being distracted by the parent. In this situation, it can be helpful to audibly explain the different chairs in the treatment room to the child and for the parents: "Here we have two special chairs in the room. You can sit on the neat up-and-down chair and your mom can sit on the magic chair there in the corner. That chair magically quiets the voice of whoever's sitting on it. This means we can talk to each other without being disturbed." It can also help to give a "strict look" in the direction of the accompanying person who is interrupting. If possible, attempt to separate the parent from their child for the treatment. If the parent will not allow it, an explanatory chat between the dentist and the parent after the treatment may help. Once again, it is useful to guide parents on what to do, either in the form of a letter (see Fig 2-1) or as text on the practice website.

Little tricks from nonverbal behavior management can be useful with very forceful parents. For example, parents can be placed lower down than the dentist on a small seat or stool in the treatment room. This enables the dentist to stay in control of the situation. When greeting parents, the dentist can deliberately move closer within their personal space. This also demonstrates superiority and taking control.

FRONT-OFFICE COMMUNICATION

Communication extends beyond the waiting room and the treatment itself. How the staff approaches scheduling also reflects the positive communication of the practice. Scheduling appointments with patients can occasionally be very difficult. If a practice has newly accepted pediatric patients, this new group of patients can pose entirely new challenges for the practice team. For mothers of babies, arranging and arriving punctually for appointments is undoubtedly a challenge. Flexibility in scheduling and accommodating the realities of life with an infant or toddler will go a long way toward keeping your patients calm and relaxed. Furthermore, morning or early afternoon appointments are generally best for children, but of course they are not always possible because of parents' working hours. Keeping in mind children's compliance, however, it is entirely reasonable to give priority to these appointments and communicate that to the parents.

It is also helpful for the front office staff to ask patients to arrive 10 minutes early for appointments. This gives the child some time to get used to the environment, to play a little, and thus to relax. In the meantime, parents can fill out the medical history form or any other necessary documentation. Furthermore, if the staff member garners any personal information when scheduling the appointment with the parents, this can be used for an individual welcome. This creates trust in the child and the parents.

REFERENCES

1. Mostofsky DI, Fortune F. Behavioral Dentistry, ed 2. Ames, IA: John Wiley & Sons, 2014.

2. Müller EM, Hasslinger Y. Sprechen Sie schon Kind?: Prophylaxe auf Augenhöhe. Berlin: Quintessenz, 2016.

3. Kossak HC, Zehner G. Hypnose beim Kinder-Zahnarzt. Verhaltensführung und Kommunikation. Heidelberg: Springer, 2011.

4. Atzlinger F. Kinderhypnose in der Zahnheilkunde. Diplomarbeit. Universität Budapest, Fakultät für Zahnmedizin, 2008. http://www.zahn1.at/service/downloads?file=files/ assets/content/Download/ DiplomarbeitKinderhypnoseinderZahnmedizinges.pdf. Accessed 26 August 2017.

5. Goho C. „Top 10" der Fehler im Umgang mit kleinen Patienten. ZWP online, 28.02.2011. http://www. zwp-online.info/zwpnews/wirtschaft-und-recht/patienten/top-10-der-fehlerim-umgang-mit-kleinen-patienten. Accessed 26 October 2018.

6. Zehner G. (Hrsg.) Quick Time Trance und Hypnopunktur, 2004. http://www.kinderzahnarzt-praxis.info/ app/download/5872895961/QuickTimeTrance+und+Hypnopunktur. pdf?t=1359880533. Accessed 2 December 2016.

7. Goho C. Die erfolgreiche Behandlung von Kindern. ZMK 2011;27(12):778-782. http:// www.zmk-aktuell.de/fachgebiete/kinderzahnheilkunde/story/die-erfolgreiche-behandlung-von-kindern_595. html. Accessed 2 December 2016.

8. Goho C. Erfolge und Misserfolge in der Kinderzahnheilkunde; Fortbildungsveranstaltung der LZÄK Sachsen, Dresden, 2011.

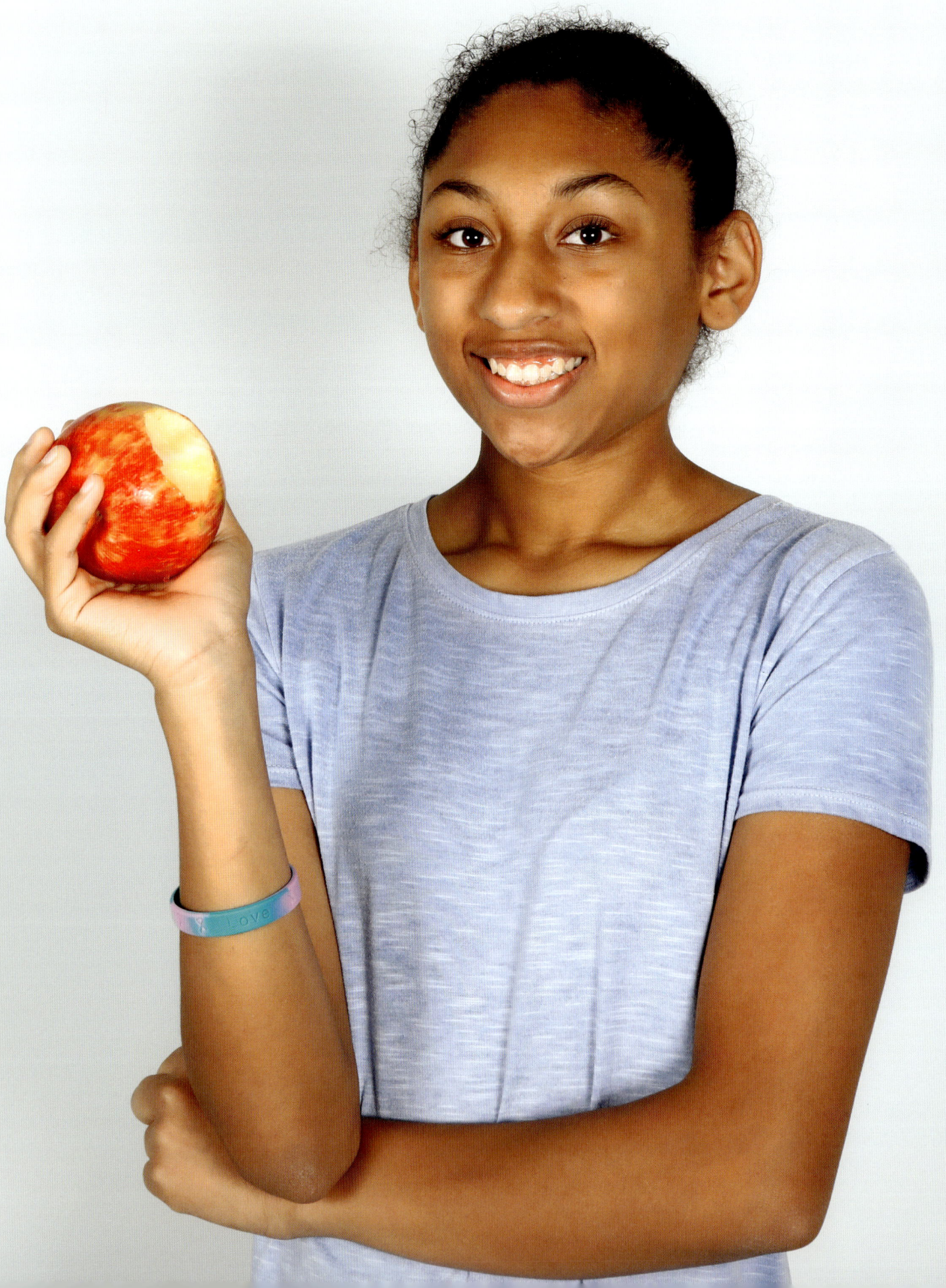

3

EDUCATING PARENTS: ORAL HYGIENE AND PROPHYLAXIS

This chapter briefly addresses issues that, based on experience, frequently preoccupy parents and which they often ask about in the explanatory discussion with their dentist. First and foremost among these is oral hygiene and prophylaxis. Parents want to know what they should be doing to prevent caries. That being said, not all parents are as motivated as the next, so we as pediatric dentists need to do our best to advocate for the oral health of our young patients.

"The older the children, the greater the worries."

ANONYMOUS

ORAL HYGIENE

There is a great deal of uncertainty among parents about oral hygiene for babies and infants. The most common elements of uncertainty include when to start oral hygiene, when and what kind of toothpaste to use, and what to do if the child struggles. It is our job to give parents answers and encourage them. This section includes tips about oral hygiene, divided into age groups.

Infants and toddlers (0–3 years)

Brushing the teeth often works well in babies without any problems. They open their mouths as a reflex when lying on their backs in a slightly over-stretched position and, as babies will explore everything with their mouths in the oral phase, a toothbrush can be a welcome diversion. Babies and infants can either be laid on the lap with their head on their parent's knees (Fig 3-1a) or on a changing table so that the parent can brush their teeth (Figs 3-1b and 3-1c).

Unfortunately, this phase comes to an end with some children or there are phases when oral hygiene is more difficult to carry out. Then parents all report the same thing: the little ones cry, resist, and thrash about. We should encourage parents in these phases to press on caringly but consistently with what daily oral hygiene involves. In the author's opinion, giving up and

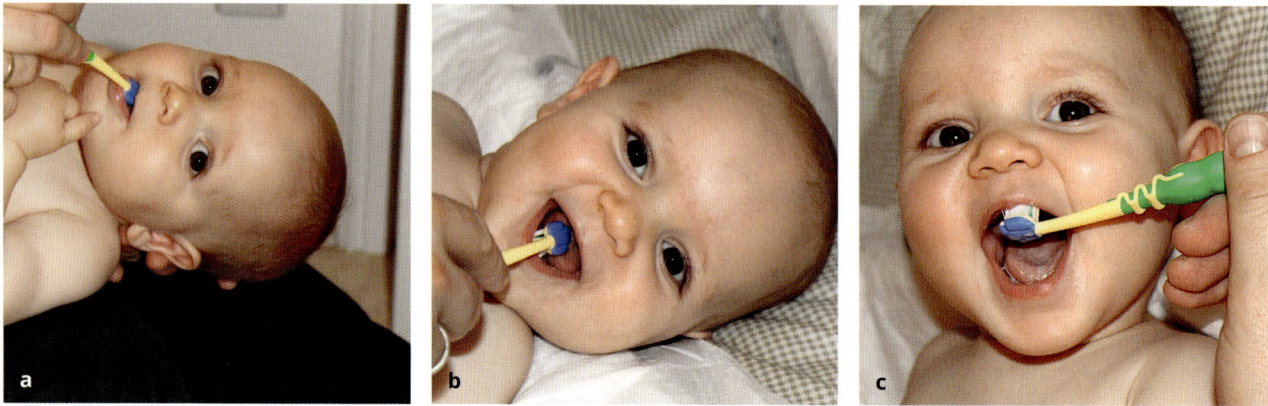

Fig 3-1 Infant tooth brushing. *(a)* The child lies on the parent's lap. With this positioning, really good brushing can be done, especially with little children. *(b and c)* Brushing an 8-month-old baby's teeth on a changing table.

skipping brushing cannot and must not be an option. We can be supportive with tips to simplify brushing and prevent possible refusal:

- First, parents can naturally get babies used to mommy and daddy wanting to take a look in their mouth. Using fun gloves specifically designed for this purpose, they can massage the alveolar ridge, for instance, which also helps prevent teething troubles. There are also special dental wipes with xylitol that can be used from day 1 to wipe the baby's mouth and accustom them to a routine. They taste good and reduce bacteria at the same time. The earlier children get used to it, the easier it will be to maintain this ritual.
- Babies can be given toothbrushes as marvelous teething aids to play with (under supervision, of course). As soon as the infant starts walking, they should not be allowed to walk or run around with their toothbrush in their mouth. They can suffer serious injuries when they fall.
- Once the first tooth actually erupts, it is advisable to have two toothbrushes: one to distract and occupy the child and one for the parents to brush their child's teeth.
- The teeth should be cleaned twice a day. Whether with fluoride toothpaste or without is dependent on the information provided by the parents in the fluoride history (see section "Fluorides").
- Parents should be cautious in the anterior dentition around the labial frenum. In nearly all infants this extends deeply. Hence, if parents clean the front teeth horizontally and bump up against the labial frenum, this might be painful for the child. The lift-the-lip technique can be used to avoid this. It involves gently pulling the top lip upward with one hand as the anterior teeth are being cleaned with the other hand (see Fig 3-2).
- Of course, brushing the teeth can be accompanied by singing, little hand puppets, or similar distractions. There are no limits to people's creativity.

- It is important to establish brushing as a daily ritual. The earlier and the more confidently this is achieved, the faster more difficult phases can be overcome.
- It is not about sticking to a schedule. In the author's opinion, how long it takes with babies and infants is initially of secondary importance; much more important than time is that all existing teeth are thoroughly cleaned from all sides.
- Often the first primary molar has already erupted when the primary canine starts to erupt. If the molar is brushed normally during this time, the eruption site of the canine might be painfully manipulated. For that reason, it is recommended that the primary molar be brushed crosswise.
- The author recommends brushing children's teeth while they are lying down. On the one hand you have better lighting for the maxillary arch and therefore a better view, and on the other hand this position is a good desensitizing method for future visits to the dentist.

WHEN BRUSHING IS A STRUGGLE

At routine checkups, many parents report that brushing their child's teeth is a daily struggle and they are helplessly seeking tips and tricks to avoid a "wrestling match." What worked entirely fine when the child was an infant has suddenly become an ordeal for all concerned. Parents do not always manage to motivate their little ones to brush or have their teeth brushed with patience and fun by including play. Especially with the youngest children, discussions or positive reinforcement with different reward systems are only possible to a limited extent.

Nonetheless, a solution must be found, because not brushing for days or weeks is not an option in terms of the child's well-being and oral health. The solution is simple: Parents just have to persevere. The more calmly and confidently parents act, the quicker this period of refusal from children is over. Refusal to brush may be a child's way of expressing desire for independence, which can turn other everyday situations (eg, diaper changing, hair washing, nail cutting, or buckling up in the car) into minor challenges. It is important for parents to understand that this autonomy phase is a completely normal developmental step after the first birthday. It is crucial that children get plenty of praise when they cooperate. This daily ritual does not have to be a struggle. It must be made clear to parents that they alone (and not the child) have to decide what is necessary for their child's health. If parents cannot manage to brush their infants' teeth for as long as a minute, how is a dentist meant to carry out a filling treatment?

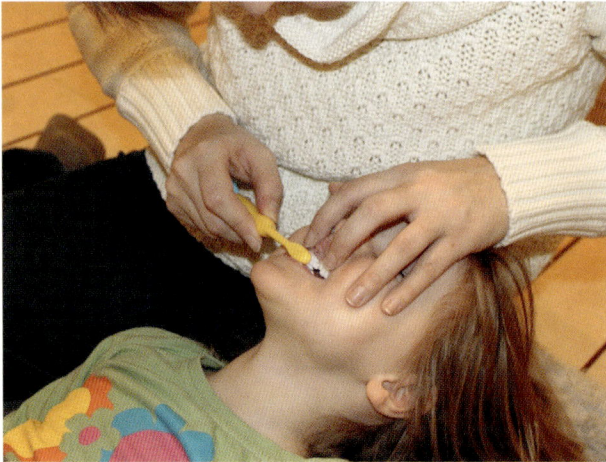

Fig 3-2 Lift-the-lip technique for atraumatic cleaning of the labial surfaces of the maxillary anterior teeth.

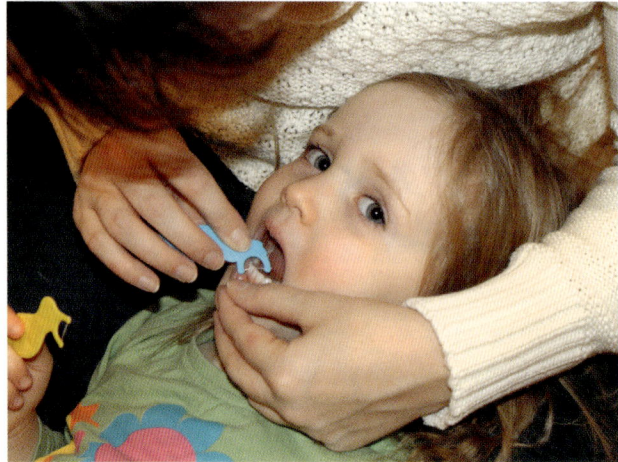

Fig 3-3 Dental floss is important if there is crowding, especially once molar eruption is completed.

Preschoolers and kindergartners (3–6 years)

Children of this age group will also have phases now and again when brushing is difficult. The cause of caries can easily be explained in an age-appropriate way to this age group—unlike babies—by using stories; it can also be made clear why cleaning their teeth is so important. This is the perfect time to institute sticker charts at home for positive reinforcement. This is a very good way of tackling difficult times and establishing daily oral hygiene as a positive way to close the day. A few more tips:

- With little children it is advisable to do follow-up brushing as the parent. Most toddlers and young children will want to brush their teeth themselves, but they do not have the dexterity or patience to do the job well. The lift-the-lip technique can still be used with this age group to atraumatically clean the anterior teeth (Fig 3-2). Regardless of whether a manual or electric toothbrush is used for follow-up brushing, ultimately only one thing counts: getting rid of the plaque! For the same reasons as mentioned earlier, it is recommended that the teeth are brushed while the child is lying down.
- Dental floss should be used for the interdental spaces in mouths with crowding and a complete dentition. There are child-themed floss holders for this purpose, which make it easy for flossing to become part of the routine (Fig 3-3).
- Parents should make sure their children have a mirror in the bathroom at the right height for them to be able to see themselves. Parents are often unaware that it is helpful for little ones to see themselves when brushing.
- On the question of whether a manual toothbrush or an electric toothbrush is better, the author recommends choosing the one where the motivation of the child is highest. It is important that children are shown the correct brushing technique for their toothbrush and that they are regularly checked to make sure that they are using it

Fig 3-4 Illustration of plaque-disclosing solution that turns plaque pink for easy visualization. (Reprinted from Terry DA. What's in Your Mouth? Chicago: Quintessence, 2013.)

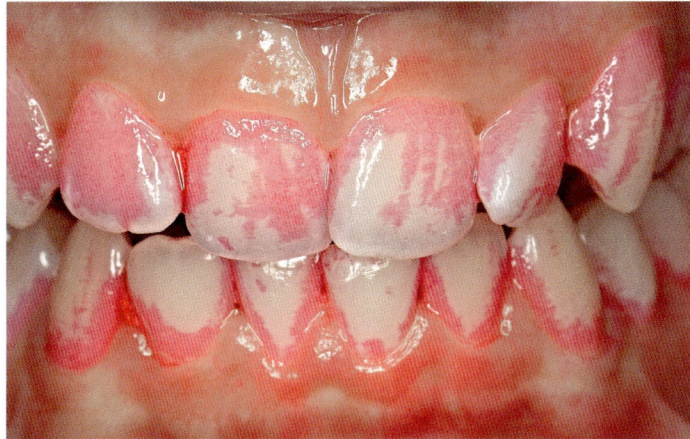

correctly. The author has also found that a constant change between manual and electric toothbrush usually results in a poorer cleaning result.

Schoolchildren (6+ years)

Many parents think that once their child starts school, oral hygiene is now a given. But that is not the case. Parents should perform follow-up cleaning of their children's teeth until the child has reached the age of 9 or 10 years. Only then are their fine motor skills so fully developed that they are largely able to do brushing at home by themselves. In the individual prophylaxis sessions at the dentist's office, specific brushing training can be performed, and again it is necessary to decide which is more appropriate for the patient: a manual or an electric toothbrush. At home parents can continually check the success of brushing with staining solutions or tablets (Fig 3-4). Visual feedback is far more successful with children than lengthy explanations.

Parents also need to be made aware of the eruption of the first and second permanent molars because no primary tooth will fall out prior to their eruption. It is very important to brush these permanent teeth crosswise during their long eruption phase because the bristles of the toothbrush will not reach their surface if the tooth has not yet reached the occlusal level.

Teenagers

In this sometimes very tricky phase when teenagers are resistant to advice, it can occasionally be very difficult to motivate patients. Good oral hygiene is crucial, especially for children with braces. If the oral hygiene is poor and the child is wearing braces, then the orthodontist should consider taking them off. Besides that, parents often have to be reminded to come back to the family dentist after orthodontic therapy. Many parents think that the orthodontist also takes care of the prophylaxis, but that is not the case.

Many parents come into the practice with the words "Please have a serious word with my child. He or she won't brush." The author refuses to do so in her role as a dental practitioner. It is not our job to raise our patients but to motivate them through positive reinforcement. What is the point of giving patients a good talking-to every 6 months if oral hygiene at home goes down the drain in between? This is why it is important to get the parents on board as allies during this phase. Regular individual prophylaxis measures and, if necessary, professional teeth cleaning can prevent dental and periodontal diseases in this phase of life. The highest priority, however, is to remotivate parents and adolescents so that oral hygiene at home is ensured between recall appointments.

PROPHYLAXIS

It is essential when treating pediatric patients to address the cause of caries and, ideally, eliminate it completely. Pediatric dentistry is not just a symptomatic "drill and fill" procedure but far more than that. Because each child is different, caries is multifactorial, and there is no panacea that works for every patient, we need to actively seek out discussion with our pediatric patients and their parents, reconsider our strategies, remotivate both child and parent, reassess our approaches, and, to the best of our knowledge and belief, choose and adopt an individual prophylaxis strategy for each particular patient. After all, what works wonderfully for one patient may fail completely with the next.

A huge range of prophylactic measures and products are available to us (dietary and drinking advice, professional tooth cleaning, at-home hygiene instructions, sealants, fluorides, etc), and it is our job to make use of these options in an individualized way according to the patient's needs. While many of the elements of dental prophylaxis are performed by dental hygienists or dental assistants, we as dentists have the responsibility to ensure that parents and children are continually remotivated and informed. We have to decide on and arrange regular recall intervals. It is proven that practices with a functioning recall and prophylaxis system have decreased incidence of caries and improved satisfaction among patients, not to mention that a well-implemented recall system is economically viable. Especially for families with difficult social or personal circumstances, it is extremely important to secure a recall schedule. Often times these children must be given extra instruction and motivation for carrying out their own oral hygiene because these steps are not being implemented rigorously by their parents. Unfortunately, caries is still a social condition.

Special equipment or materials are not necessarily required for prophylaxis in childhood. It is more important to get the parents on board and simplify and shorten the existing prophylactic steps so that they succeed in a child-appropriate way. This requires a colleague with a knack for dealing with children as well as some specific further training in this field. Prophylaxis for our young patients should be fun, pain-free, and not take too long.

TIP FOR PROPHYLAXIS WITH CHILDREN

It is important, especially in pediatric dentistry, to make compromises without losing sight of the final goal. If a child does not want to have his or her teeth cleaned, it often works if the assistant uses their electric toothbrush instead of the prophy angle. Even the child's own toothpaste can be used to clean the teeth. The main goal is that the plaque is removed so that the fluoride varnish can be applied and work. There are also inexpensive, child-friendly materials that improve compliance (eg, prophy angles that look like animals, flavored fluoride varnish, colored gloves, masks with painted faces). Sometimes it's the little things that make all the difference.

Talking to parents

Sometimes the discussion with parents is a greater challenge than treating their children. This is partly due to a generation of parents who are confused, for instance, because of the widely varying sources of information or who increasingly question our scientifically based measures. Another factor is that the timing of the visit to the dentist may be unfavorable—for instance, if a strong and acute need for treatment already exists.

It is not always easy to convey sometimes very extensive information to parents in a focused, concise, and understandable manner so that they are able to follow the advice when they get home. A lot of parents only remember the last three sentences of a far-ranging discussion with the dentist. Why is that?

On the one hand, a visit to the dentist is stressful for many parents. Not only because they have to get one or more children there on time and they have to cope with the waiting time and any boredom that may be building up, but because visiting the dentist is associated with stress and anxiety for many parents themselves, and now they are managing the anxiety of their children as well. All these factors can diminish parents' attention during an extensive explanatory discussion. This is why it is so important to keep the discussion brief and individualized, for example, based on the completed medical history form. A good method is to check the completed medical form for risk factors (eg, frequent juice drinking or oral hygiene that is performed only by the child) and mark them before we retrieve the child from the waiting room. Then we can concentrate on the risk factors and age-appropriate facts to discuss with the parents rather than telling them information they do not need at this point. The main goal should be to gain the loyalty of future parents, young parents with their babies, and the children themselves right from the very beginning in order to accompany them into a healthy life. Children are not able to take responsibility for their own oral hygiene—we have to get the parents on board from the very beginning. This is the only way we can monitor and influence children's oral health, which is an integral part of any healthy physical development.

Now and then parents are profoundly confused because they get contradictory advice from midwives, pediatricians, dentists, and, last but not least, from the Internet.

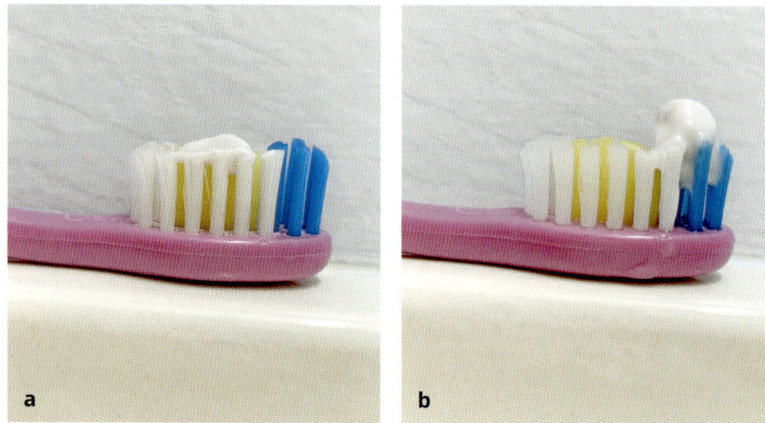

Fig 3-5 Examples of a smear (a) and pea-sized amount (b) of toothpaste.

This is why it is all the more important for the dental team to give consistent advice as the authority responsible for dental health.

Fluorides

Fluorides are the most important pillar of caries prevention. They are safe in the concentrations we use and prescribe, their action has been repeatedly proved scientifically, and in our dental practices we see the positive effects of prophylaxis and treatment with fluorides every day. In the dental practice, the medical history form should include questions about possible sources of fluoride (toothpaste, supplements prescribed by a pediatrician, mouthwashes, fluoride water intake) and the frequency of their use. Parents must be told about the consequences of avoiding fluoridation (increased caries risk) and about the consequences of overdosing (fluorosis).

The American Academy of Pediatrics recommends that fluoridated toothpaste be used for all children starting at tooth eruption.[1] Only a smear (the size of a grain of rice) should be used to the age of 3 years, after which a pea-sized amount is appropriate until age 6 (Fig 3-5). These small amounts may reduce the risk of fluorosis, according to the American Academy of Pediatric Dentistry (AAPD).[2] The teeth should be brushed twice a day. Furthermore, professionally applied fluoride varnish is recommended every 3 to 6 months starting at tooth emergence.

Water fluoridation levels are also important. Each city, state, and county all have different levels of fluoride in the water, so it is advisable to contact your state or city water supply to check these levels. If the water is not fluoridated or insufficiently fluoridated, or even if the child simply does not drink it, fluoride supplements are recommended (Table 3-1). Fluoridated water should be used to mix formula for babies who are bottle-fed. The recommendations for fluoride administration at home and in the dental practice for high-risk children are given in chapter 7.

If parents simply want to brush fluoride-free, they must be told about the increased risk of caries. It is indeed a fact that thorough oral hygiene and adequate caries prevention

TABLE 3-1 Dietary fluoride supplementation schedule based on water fluoridation levels

Age	< 0.3 ppm F	0.3–0.6 ppm F	> 0.6 ppm F
Birth to 6 months	0	0	0
6 months to 3 years	0.25 mg	0	0
3 to 6 years	0.5 mg	0.25 mg	0
6 to at least 16 years	1 mg	0.5 mg	0

are possible even with fluoride-free toothpaste. As far as the author is concerned, there is no use trying to convince absolute fluoride opponents. However, it should be made absolutely clear that other caries-preventive measures (especially reducing daily sugar intake) must be taken to successfully prevent caries.

Along with careful oral hygiene, reducing sugar consumption is the only really efficient measure in prophylaxis without fluorides. Admittedly, parents easily underestimate what is meant by the term "sugar reduction." The World Health Organization recommends maximum daily consumption of free sugars of 10% relative to total calorie intake. To achieve caries reduction, a reduction to 5% is probably required; that is equivalent to a total sugar quantity of 15 g for children.[3] For comparison, one can of Coke contains approximately 35 g sugar, and one serving of the average breakfast cereal we find on most tables has about 10 g of sugar. These figures can make it clear to parents how difficult it is to reduce the quantities of sugar consumed so sharply that a caries-preventive effect is really noticeable. In other words, caries prophylaxis is possible without fluoride, but it is very difficult for most of the families we treat.

GRINDING TEETH

Many parents will tell you about the grinding sounds coming from their children, primarily at night. Prevalence rates in the literature range from 6% to 50%, which illustrates the inconsistent nature of the studies on this subject.[4] Some natural abrasion of the primary teeth is physiologic as part of the dynamic growth and development process and may even be necessary to ensure proper jaw growth and physiologic alignment of the 6-year molars.[5]

In extremely rare cares, however, primary teeth exhibit levels of attrition that require treatment. In a review, Restrepo et al wrote that the available literature did not support demands to treat bruxism in children.[6] Nevertheless, there are studies that provide evidence of pathologic causes of nocturnal bruxism. In a study from 2009, Serra-Negra et al discovered that children exhibiting certain personality traits (a high degree of responsibility and neuroticism) have a higher rate of nocturnal bruxism.[7] DiFrancesco et al reported that children's nocturnal tooth grinding significantly improved after tonsillectomy and adenoidectomy.[8] This shows that nocturnal grinding can also be caused by myofunctional imbalances; the reasons for this can be various (eg, mouth breathing, adenoids, tongue-tie, etc) and must be examined.

If the levels of attrition are extremely high, dentists should carry out myofunctional diagnostics, check for tongue-tie, and, if necessary, consult an ENT (ear, nose, and throat) physician in an interdisciplinary approach to exclude any narrowing of the upper airways. Behavioral therapy measures for older children (stress reduction) are also a possibility. It is important to understand that tooth grinding in the permanent dentition can no longer be classified as a physiologic part of the growth process.

TEETHING

Teething is a common concern for parents because it results in lack of sleep for the whole family as well as various side effects during the developmental stage. While infants are teething, parents often report issues such as red cheeks, raised temperature or fever, diarrhea, tearfulness, increased salivation, nonspecific skin rash, increased cough, and general clinginess or whiny behavior. There are various measures that parents can take to relieve their child's teething pains and these unpleasant side effects. Parents are often grateful for tips because they lessen their own sense of helplessness in dealing with an overtired, unhappy baby.

As a preventive measure, parents can regularly massage their infant's gums with special teething gloves and mittens. Because this oral phase begins within the first year of a child's life, most infants will allow these sorts of manipulations in the mouth without difficulty. These aids ensure that the gingiva is well perfused and, as a positive side effect, babies become accustomed early to oral hygiene rituals they will experience later.

Depending on the child's age, parent preference, and the severity of the problems, mechanical aids or pain-relieving products can be used to soothe teething infants. Growth spurts are often accompanied by tooth eruption, which makes it difficult to differentiate which area of development is the source of discomfort for the child.

Teething aids

Teething aids such as a chilled teething ring or washcloth can provide relief. When using teething rings, it is important to make sure the products are free of toxins. In tests, a few products have been found to contain phthalates (plasticizers); these certainly have no place inside a child's mouth. Teething rings do not belong in the freezer because they will become too hard, potentially causing injury to the oral mucosa. Furthermore, freezing makes teething rings porous more quickly. The rings should be cleaned regularly under hot water. When using teething rings, parents should make sure they are not used habitually but in a focused, restrictive way and when required. Otherwise, they can prevent the child from maturing in a myofunctional sense.[5]

Local pain relievers

Many parents will ask about medicinal remedies for teething. While there are products available for such purpose, the US Food and Drug Administration (FDA) and the AAPD warn against their use due to their potential for toxicity.[9,10] Further, pain-relieving teething gels that contain lidocaine or benzocaine are not recommended because they have only a limited duration of action, are hard to dose correctly, and most of the product is swallowed. A statement from the FDA in 2014 clearly advised against the use of 2% lidocaine in teething infants. The FDA had reviewed 22 cases in which serious medical incidents occurred in children in connection with lidocaine and reported convulsions, brain damage, and heart problems as consequences of overdosing. In addition, the FDA had already published a warning against benzocaine in 2011 because, when used topically, there were rare cases of life-threatening methemoglobinemia.[11] As well as local anesthetics, the products contain preservatives with an appreciable potential for allergization, which argues against their use in children.

Systemic pain relievers

If teething aids do not work and there is a need for pain relief, then acetaminophen and ibuprofen are perfectly suitable for the systemic treatment of teething troubles. These oral analgesics are even endorsed by the AAPD.[10] The relevant dosage instructions should be strictly followed. Administration of these analgesics will quickly and reliably get rid of pain for several hours. Ibuprofen additionally has an anti-inflammatory effect, and acetaminophen is antipyretic. Unlike topical gels, their systemic use eliminates pain for longer and more reliably, and precise dosing is guaranteed.

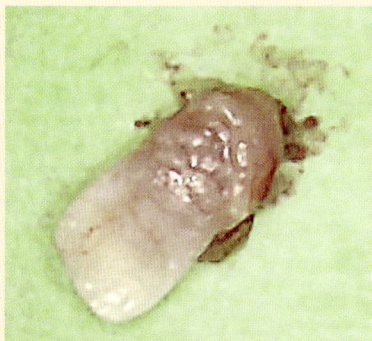

Fig 3-6 Removed natal tooth. The mother attended the practice with the 5-day-old patient. Both mandibular lateral incisors were already present at birth, and one had already been removed by the midwife in the hospital. Removal of this tooth was done with a small bone nibbling forceps without local anesthetic. The newborn slept through the entire treatment.

NATAL TEETH

The average age when the first primary teeth erupt is around 6 months. In isolated cases, eruption can occur in the first 4 weeks of life (neonatal teeth) or, by contrast, not until after the child's first birthday. There are also rare cases of babies who are born with teeth. These natal teeth are mainly mandibular incisors and less commonly the maxillary incisors. In 95% of cases, it is not a matter of supernumerary tooth germs.[12] As the roots are not developed or only in a very rudimentary way, the teeth are usually very loose, making it necessary to remove them (Fig 3-6). Their extraction will prevent them from being aspirated or becoming an obstacle to nursing or bottle feeding.

⟶

Occasionally, they are also the reason for small mucosal lesions appearing at the tip of the tongue. Removal is done either with a swab or small bone nibbling forceps if the tiny teeth cannot be properly grabbed with just a swab. A topical anesthetic can be applied but is not necessarily required. If neonatal teeth are present that are firmly in place and are causing no discomfort, they can be left as they are.

PACIFIER USE AND THUMB SUCKING

One of the trickiest issues to navigate in pediatric dentistry is children sucking on their thumb and/or a pacifier. It starts with the question "What's better?" The great advantage of a pacifier is surely that it can easily be removed when weaning the baby off it; the drawback is that it gets used more intensively than the thumb during the period of use.[13] On the other hand, the thumb is more readily available to children than a pacifier and, unlike a pacifier, it obviously can never be taken away by a parent. Although in most cases the thumb is used for less time over the day, infants are still weaned off it much later, which can cause a number of malformations. Among 2- to 5-year-olds, thumb sucking is the most significant etiologic factor for an anterior open bite. This open bite can be symmetric or, less favorably, asymmetric. An open bite can cause speech disorders, esthetic impairments, changes in the swallowing pattern, myofunctional disorders, and difficulties in biting food with the anterior teeth.[14] Obviously these anomalies can equally be caused by prolonged use of a pacifier. In answer to the question of which is preferred, use of a pacifier still tends to be preferred over thumb sucking. Regarding daily use of a pacifier, Dr Andrea Thumeyer wrote, "Use a pacifier as sparingly as a medicine."[15]

Parents often ask whether their dentist can recommend a certain brand of pacifier to minimize these potential problems. In the author's experience, this choice only partly lies in the hands of the parents because not every child will accept every pacifier. Pacifiers with a very narrow or soft shaft are usually recommended. However, all pacifiers (whether or not they are ergonomically designed) hold the tongue away from its physiologic resting position on the palate, which inevitably will lead to malformations if the pacifier is used too frequently and/or over a long period of time. Far more important than the shape or brand is instructing parents on restricting and limiting the use of pacifiers and when to begin the weaning process. Parents should continue using smaller pacifiers because the larger the pacifier, the greater the risk of malformation. Furthermore, heavy pacifier chains should be avoided because they increase the weight of the pacifier and also the forces acting on the teeth and surrounding structures. Furtenbach answers the question about the best pacifier with: "The best pacifier is the one you don't give to your child."[5]

Another key question is obviously when to wean children off pacifiers or thumb sucking. With regard to pacifiers, Schopf writes, "if weaning off this habit takes place by the age of 3 years, there is a significant and age-dependent increasing trend to avoidance of an open bite."[13] Weaning should thus be started around the child's second birthday. From an orthodontist's point of view, the pacifier should then be "disappeared." For speech therapists, the optimum time to begin weaning is when the child starts to talk (varies between individuals, but generally between 7 and 12 months). If children are weaned off their pacifier too late, there is a risk that an open bite of the primary teeth will persist through to the mixed dentition. This is because, when they have been weaned off a pacifier, the tip of the tongue likes to occupy the space of the pacifier and the bite is no longer able to close.

Several possible ways of weaning off a pacifier are described in the literature. Ultimately, however, success depends entirely on the parents' persistence. It is helpful to link giving up the pacifier to a special day or holiday such as Christmas or Easter. Parents can persuade their child to give up their pacifier to a younger sibling or family member. If the parent explains that the younger child now needs the pacifier, the child may feel more inclined to part with it, now that they are more "grown up." Another way to wean children off pacifiers is to send the pacifier to a "pacifier fairy" or hang it on a "pacifier tree." A pacifier tree (sometimes referred to as a *binky tree*) is a tree that is full of old pacifiers that children have given up; these trees are usually in large cities. Parents can also trim the teat gradually or puncture it with holes to make sucking unattractive to the child. This approach works very well too.

It is much more difficult to wean children off thumb sucking. The average age when children stop sucking their thumb is 3.8 years.[16] When children are aged between 0 and 3 years, it is a good idea for parents to praise them when they do not suck on anything (positive reinforcement). Between 3 and 5 years, behavioral therapy can be attempted with the dentist's support. In doing this, the dentist should act as an ally on the side of the child, motivating rather than scolding. Parents can also put bandages on the thumb that gets sucked. These would come off if sucked, so parents can give their child a little prize if the bandage survives the day unharmed. The process, like weaning off any other sucking habit, should be accompanied by plenty of positive reinforcement. Commercial thumb-sucking liquids as a form of a negative reinforcement should not be used and have not proved effective in everyday practice. Binding fingers or hands is also counterproductive. For intractable cases, the use of devices such as an oral screen or therapeutic methods such as the myofunctional therapy described above should be considered.[17]

CARIES DUE TO BREASTFEEDING

Breastfeeding is best for mother and baby in many ways. From the dental and speech therapy perspective, breastfeeding is the best form of myofunctional and hence orthodontic prophylaxis. It strengthens the entire oral and perioral musculature, trains lip closure, encourages the sensitivity of the oral cavity, reinforces nasal breathing, prepares the tongue and lips for eventual articulation, strengthens the mother-baby bond, and promotes the baby's socioemotional development. The latter also has a beneficial effect on later speech development.[5] Therefore, pediatric dentists should definitely encourage their pregnant patients to breastfeed their children when asked for their opinion. Of course it is the individual decision of a mother if and how long she wants to breastfeed her child according to her own circumstances in life. It is your responsibility to address the scientific basis of why breastfeeding is recommended, but it is always best to approach this conversation with sensitivity.

In the dental context, prolonged and high-frequency breastfeeding at night has been viewed critically. While breast milk on its own does not increase the risk for early childhood caries (ECC), together with other carbohydrates, it has been classified as highly cariogenic in in vitro studies.[18] Studies further prove that breastfeeding beyond 2 years markedly increases the risk of caries.[19] However, several studies have reported that it is not the duration of breastfeeding that increases the risk of caries but instead the way in which breastfeeding is performed, specifically in frequent, short nighttime feeds.[20,21] A meta-analysis from 2015 concluded that children who are breastfed beyond 12 months have a higher risk of caries and that the risk was also increased in this group if they were breastfed more frequently at night.[22] As such, parents must be made aware that very frequent, short, nonnutritive nighttime breastfeeding episodes when primary teeth are present are indisputably a major risk factor and can be a contributory cause of ECC. But why is that?

Caries is a multifactorial disease that can be influenced by many factors. One cannot say definitively that breastfeeding will certainly cause caries if a baby is breastfed beyond 12 months of life. Many other factors play a role here. We pediatric dentists often see children in our practice who are breastfed far beyond that age and show no lesions whatsoever. But it is also an undisputed fact that very common, short, nonnutritive nocturnal breastfeeding episodes with existing primary teeth can be a major risk factor contributing to caries. We also see these patients again and again. The following factors are responsible for the increased caries risk:

- Oral hygiene is not possible at night.
- Salivation is strongly reduced, therefore only an insufficient buffering of the decreasing pH value is taking place.
- Breast milk contains approximately 7.2% lactose (for comparison, cow's milk contains approximately 4.5%).
- Because it contains only small amounts of caries-inhibiting components such as calcium and phosphate, breast milk can reduce the intraoral pH below 5.5, which leads to a demineralization of the primary tooth enamel.[20]

Short and frequent nightly breastfeeding episodes beyond the first birthday of the child are usually more of a sleeping or calming aid that can be viewed independently of food intake. This nonnutritive sucking pattern is entirely different from a normal, nutritive breastfeeding sucking mechanism. It is characterized by a high sucking frequency but a low sucking activity, which means that only so-called "foremilk" (ie, the milk produced in the first nursing phase) is produced. In this milk, the lactose content is in aqueous solution, and thus available for bacteria to be metabolized, and rinses around the maxillary incisors.[20] During nutritive breastfeeding, children suck much more vigorously, which leads to the production of so-called "hindmilk." While this hindmilk contains the same amount of lactose as the foremilk, in hindmilk this lactose content is bound to fat molecules, so the harmful effect in the mouth is directly avoided because there is no enzyme in the mouth that is able to split fat components. The lactose content is only split off once it is in the stomach. In addition, during a nutritive sucking pattern the milk does not touch the teeth but is expressed at the palate and swallowed. With all these factors, comfort nocturnal breastfeeding can indeed be a caries risk factor. Furtenbach also wrote that "the breast is not to be used as a pacifier" because the physiologic oral flora needs rest.[5] This is exactly the crucial point.

When highly frequent and prolonged breastfeeding is identified as a caries risk factor in a patient, we should encourage parents to reduce nighttime nursing, to quench baby's thirst with water if possible, and to find ways to make it easier for baby to fall asleep without breastfeeding, primarily by establishing a different bedtime ritual that does not involve breastfeeding. Infants who are used to only falling asleep at the breast obviously find it harder to settle down again without the breast in occurring waking phases. Therefore, mothers are advised not to let their babies fall asleep at their breast from the age of about 6 months but rather to breastfeed, then brush the teeth before continuing to the rest of the bedtime ritual (singing, looking at books, etc). Moreover, we should check for lip and tongue-ties that might be an influencing factor as well. The question of caries risk is less about "how long" and more about "what form" breastfeeding takes.

It is important to discuss this highly sensitive subject with parents calmly and nonjudgmentally. Pediatric dentists, in particular, are often reproached for advising against breastfeeding. Especially in view of the multifactorial etiologic model of caries and the many advantages that breastfeeding affords mother and child, it is extremely important for our profession to encourage breastfeeding when appropriate. After all, socioeconomic status is more important as a caries risk factor than the source of a baby's nutrition.[23]

While the decision about the duration of breastfeeding lies with each mother herself, all nursing mothers should be made aware of the subject and should be instructed on how to ensure good oral hygiene in their infant. We dentists should and indeed must contribute to this part of the parents' education.

Bottle caries

Bottle-fed or formula-fed babies are just as susceptible to ECC from nighttime feedings or too-frequent "snacking" on the bottle during the day. A baby should never be sent to bed with a bottle of milk for nighttime soothing, and a bottle should not be used as a pacifier during the day. While these practices may seem convenient for parents to avoid nighttime wakings or fussy babies, it's the frequency of feeding that can become a major risk factor for ECC.

The same is true for solid foods. Children do not have to eat or chew something throughout the whole day. It should be made clear to parents that eating and drinking should be offered numerous times throughout the day but should not be something that is carried out constantly. The oral flora needs rest for the saliva to buffer the decreasing intraoral pH and therefore to stop demineralization of the primary teeth.

DIETARY AND DRINKING HABITS

What children drink

The most important thing about dietary and drinking advice in relation to ECC is certainly educating parents about drinks and the frequency of consumption. Parents are sometimes concerned about how much liquid intake their child should have every day. As a result, they often give their children juice just to make sure they get enough to drink. But a glass of apple juice contains more sugar than the same amount of Coke; bearing that in mind, it is definitely not a good alternative.

In terms of whether or not children are drinking enough liquid, dentists can reassure parents that no child will voluntarily die of thirst! Children are not just taking in liquid when they drink but also nutrients in a bound form. Infants who are fully breastfed do not need any additional fluid intake. When more solid foods are introduced at about 7 months old, an additional fluid intake of approximately 200 mL/day should be provided in the form of water.[24]

Without a doubt, water is the best thirst quencher. Parents need to be told that taste is instilled or acquired in children. The sentence "My child doesn't drink water" is merely the result of wrongly acquired drinking habits based on a bad example. The effect of parents as role models in training their children's dietary and drinking habits is not to be underestimated. Flavored water is not, as many parents assume, a healthy alternative.

How they drink it

How children drink is also important. Roughly at the start of eating solids, children can learn how to drink from normal, thin-walled cups. At this age, infants cannot sit up by themselves yet, but if half-sitting with proper support for their head, they can drink out of a cup. It is entirely unnecessary to get infants accustomed to drinking from a bottle or from a training cup before transitioning to an open cup. Training cups like these prevent the development of a somatic swallowing pattern[5] and can result in myofunctional and speech issues if the immature sucking pattern persists.[25] If drinking in a sitting position is practiced, the cup should be well-filled, especially at the start because infants cannot yet tip their heads back to drink. Obviously they might spill a bit to begin with and even swallow the drink all at once, but parents will notice that drinking from a cup is a thoroughly intuitive process that children observe and imitate (Fig 3-7).

If parents prefer a training cup while on the go, those without a spout or teat attachment are suitable. There are also leak-proof screwable cups for carrying around, enabling infants to drink quite normally from the edge.

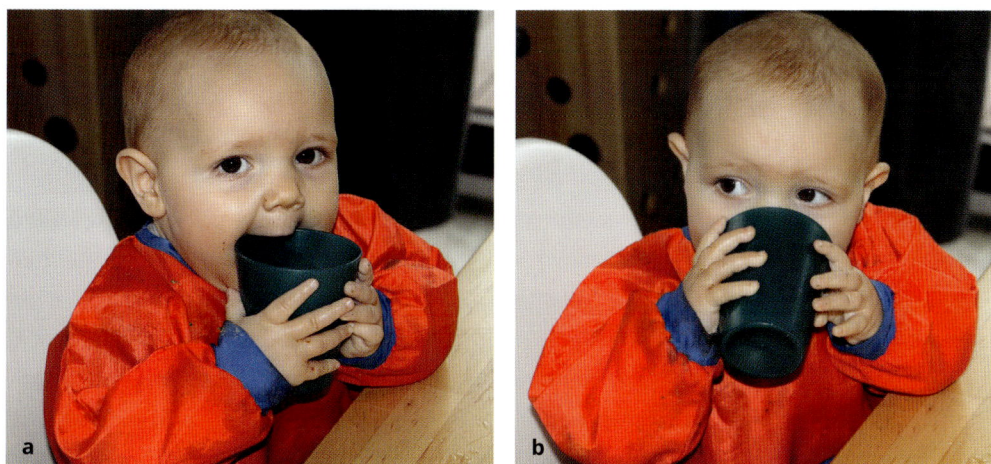

Fig 3-7 *(a and b)* Eight-month-old infant drinking from a normal, thin-walled cup.

TIPS FOR ENCOURAGING HEALTHY DRINKING HABITS

- *Water, water, and more water:* Parents greatly underestimate the erosive and cariogenic potential of juices and carbonated beverages. Children should primarily drink plain water (not flavored water).
- *Be a role model:* Mom and dad can hardly urge their child to drink water if they are drinking soda or iced tea.
- *Use a regular cup:* Sippy cups or other training cups can train the muscles improperly. Children should be introduced to a regular cup before their first birthday.
- *Bottle use:* It is extremely important not to let children constantly suck on a bottle. Even a bottle of milk or something similar as a bedtime ritual is dangerous and can lead to ECC very quickly. Children should be offered something to drink several times a day, but a bottle should not be a toy, a pacifier substitute, or a method to calm a child down.

Sugar and childhood obesity

American children consume too much sugar, and this is a leading contributing factor to childhood obesity. The US Centers for Disease Control and Prevention report childhood obesity at 18.5% in the United States (13.9% for 2- to 5-year-olds, 18.4% among 6- to 11-year-olds, and 20.6% among 12- to 19-year-olds), with greater percentages among Hispanic and non-Hispanic black populations.[26] It is becoming increasingly apparent that the assumption in recent decades that fats are largely responsible for obesity cannot really be supported. Studies show that sugar in particular has a very negative influence on the overall metabolism. Even in experiments where the total calories remained the same but the amount of sugar was reduced, positive effects such as lowered blood sugar, lowered LDL cholesterol, lowered triglycerides, improved liver function, and lowered insulin levels became apparent quickly. In addition, the subjects under a low-sugar diet reacted much more strongly to satiety stimuli. This shows that "one calorie is not equal to one calorie."[27]

Obesity and its accompanying symptoms are now among the most pressing health issues worldwide. In most cases, it is children who suffer from obesity for the rest of their lives, because, contrary to popular belief, people do not grow out of being overweight; rather it is a serious disease. While diet is not the only contributing factor to obesity, it is our responsibility as pediatric dentists to address it for the sake of our young patients' health. Specifically, we can raise parents' awareness of this subject and expose and thereby prevent possible dietary traps. These include too frequent and uncontrolled snacking between meals, portion sizes that are too big, and calorie intake that is too high (eg, when drinking smoothies or soft drinks). Parents should also be alerted to the tricks of the industry ("healthy" flavored water, extra-sweet products for children, and sweets at children's eye level at every supermarket checkout). It is up to parents to make conscious choices to limit their child's sugar intake. Of course some sweets are inevitable and perfectly fine in life, but the key is moderation.

TIPS FOR ENCOURAGING HEALTHY EATING HABITS

- *Eat meals together as a family:* It has been proven that children eat healthier when there is a dedicated meal time free of TV or other distractions.
- *Be a role model:* You cannot expect a child to eat healthily if the parent does not offer healthy choices or eats junk food themselves.
- *Timing:* Sugar-free breaks are important so that the teeth have time to remineralize and the saliva can buffer the acidic pH. Even healthy foods like fruit should be eaten in one sitting and not nibbled on throughout the day to prevent the accumulation of sugars on the teeth.
- *Natural sugar is still sugar:* Honey and other naturally sweet products are still full of sugar and should be moderated just like artificial sugars. While dried fruits can be a great snack, they are naturally sticky and adhere to the occlusal surfaces for a long time, so parents should limit their consumption.
- *It's all about moderation!*
- *Marketing to children:* Products especially designed for children usually contain up to 20% more sugar than the normal alternative. Parents need to know this.
- *Food consistency:* The consistency of food is crucial for good teeth and jaw development. Children do not need smoothies or drinkable yogurts but rather things to chew on in order to develop jaw muscles.

REFERENCES

1. American Academy of Pediatrics. AAP Recommends Fluoride to Prevent Dental Caries. https://www.aap.org/en-us/about-the-aap/aap-press-room/Pages/AAP-Recommends-Fluoride-to-Prevent-Dental-Caries.aspx. Accessed 31 January 2020.

2. American Academy of Pediatric Dentistry. Fluoride Therapy. https://www.aapd.org/media/Policies_Guidelines/BP_FluorideTherapy.pdf. Accessed 31 January 2020.

3. Schiffner U. Evidenz kariespräventiver Maßnahmen in 1. und 2. Dentition; Vortrag im Rahmen der DGKIZ-Jahrestagung 2017; Leipzig, 30.09.2017.

4. Machado E, Dal-Fabbro C, Cunali PA, Kaizer OB. Prevalence of sleep bruxism in children: A systematic review. Dental Press J Orthod 2014;19:54–61.

5. Furtenbach M, Adamer I (Hrsg.). Myofunktionelle Therapie Kompakt II: Diagnostik und Therapie. Ein Denk- und Arbeitsbuch. Vienna: Praesens Verlag, 2016.

6. Restrepo CC, Gómez S, Manrique R. Treatment of bruxism in children: A systematic review. Quintessence Int 2009;40:849–855.

7. Serra-Negra JM, Ramos-Jorge M, Flores-Mendoza CE, Paiva SM, Pordeus IA. Influence of psychosocial factors on the development of sleep bruxism among children. Int J Paediatr Dent 2009;19:309–317.

8. DiFrancesco RC, Junqueira PA, Trezza PM, de Faria ME, Frizzarini R, Zerati FE. Improvement of bruxism after T & A surgery. Int J Pediatr Otorhinolaryngol 2004;68:441–445.

9. US Food and Drug Administration. FDA Drug Safety Communication: Reports of a rare, but serious and potentially fatal adverse effect with the use of over-the-counter (OTC) benzocaine gels and liquids applied to the gums or mouth. https://www.fda.gov/drugs/drug-safety-and-availability/fda-drug-safety-communication-reports-rare-serious-and-potentially-fatal-adverse-effect-use-over. Accessed 31 January 2020.

10. American Academy of Pediatric Dentistry. Perinatal and Infant Oral Health Care. https://www.aapd.org/globalassets/media/policies_guidelines/bp_perinataloralhealthcare.pdf. Accessed 31 January 2020.

11. US Food and Drug Administration. Benzocaine and Babies: Not a Good Mix. https://www.fda.gov/ForConsumers/ConsumerUpdates/ucm306062.htm. Accessed 30 October 2015.

12. Lemos L, Shintome LK, Ramos CJ, Myaki SI. Natal and neonatal teeth. Einstein 2009;7:112–113.

13. Schopf P. Curriculum Kieferorthopädie, Band I und II. Berlin: Quintessenz, 2008.

14. Ize-Iyamu IN, Isiekwe MC. Prevalence and factors associated with anterior open bite in 2 to 5 year old children in Benin city, Nigeria. Afr Health Sci 2012;12:446–451.

15. Thumeyer A. Dauernuckeln ist schlecht für Zähne und Herz – Den Schnuller so sparsam einsetzen wie ein Medikament. Herzblatt 2014:12–13.

16. Goho C. Erfolge und Misserfolge in der Kinderzahnheilkunde; Fortbildungsveranstaltung der LZÄK Sachsen. Dresden: 2011.

17. Fuhlbrück S. Wie die Mundatmung Zunge, Zähne und Sprache beeinflusst – Erfahrungen mit der Myofunktionellen Therapie und der Körperorientierten Sprachtherapie k-o-s-t® nach Susanne Codoni, CH. Co-med 2010:1–5.

18. AAPD: Policy on Early Childhood Caries (ECC): Classifications, Consequences, and Preventive Strategies. http://www.aapd.org/media/Policies_Guidelines/P_ECCClassifications.pdf. Accessed 25 October 2017.

19. Peres KG, Nascimento GG, Peres MA, et al. Impact of prolonged breastfeeding on dental caries: A population-based birth cohort study. Pediatrics 2017;140.

20. Bissar A, Schiller P, Wolf A, Niekusch U, Schulte AG. Factors contributing to severe early childhood caries in south-west Germany. Clini Oral Investig 2014;18:1411–1418.

21. Chaffee BW, Feldens CA, Vitolo MR. Association of long-duration breastfeeding and dental caries estimated with marginal structural models. Ann Epidemiol 2014;24:448–454.

22. Tham R, Bowatte G, Dharmage SC, et al. Breastfeeding and the risk of dental caries: A systematic review and meta analysis. Acta Paediatr 2015;104:62–84.

23. Roberts GJ, Cleaton-Jones PE, Fatti LP, et al. Patterns of breast and bottle feeding and their association with dental caries in 1- to 4-year-old South African children. 1. Dental caries prevalence and experience. Community Dent Health 1993;10:405–413.

24. Koletzko B, Brönstrup A, Cremer M, et al. Säuglingsernährung und Ernährung der stillenden Mutter: Handlungsempfehlungen – Ein Konsensuspapier im Auftrag des bundesweiten Netzwerk Junge Familie. Monatsschr Kinderheilkd 2010;158:679–689.

25. Thumeyer A, Städtler A, Bolten MA, Zimmer St. Trinken aus dem offenen Becher. Zahnärztl Mitt 2011;(19):102–104.

26. Centers for Disease Control and Prevention. Childhood Obesity Facts. https://www.cdc.gov/obesity/data/childhood.html. Accessed 31 January 2020.

27. Lustig RH, Mulligan K, Noworolski SM, et al. Isocaloric fructose restriction and metabolic improvement in children with obesity and metabolic syndrome. Obesity 2016;24:453–460.

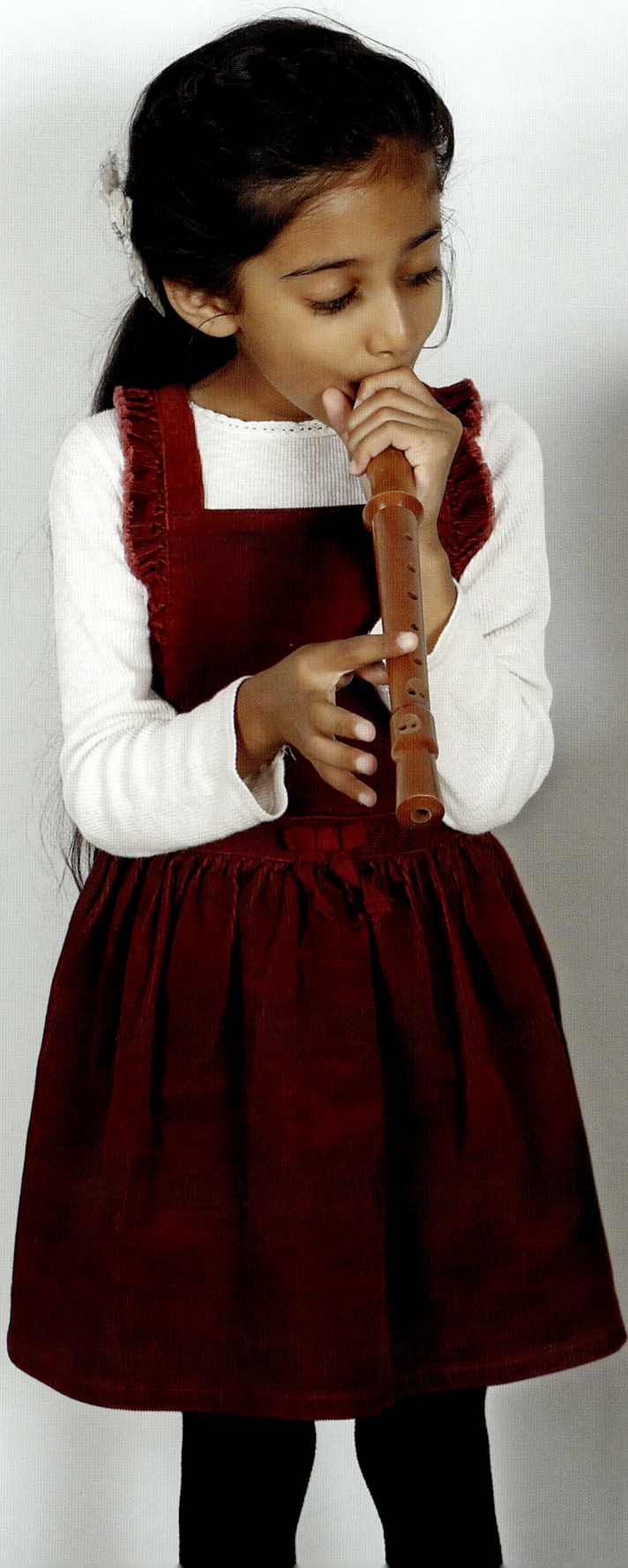

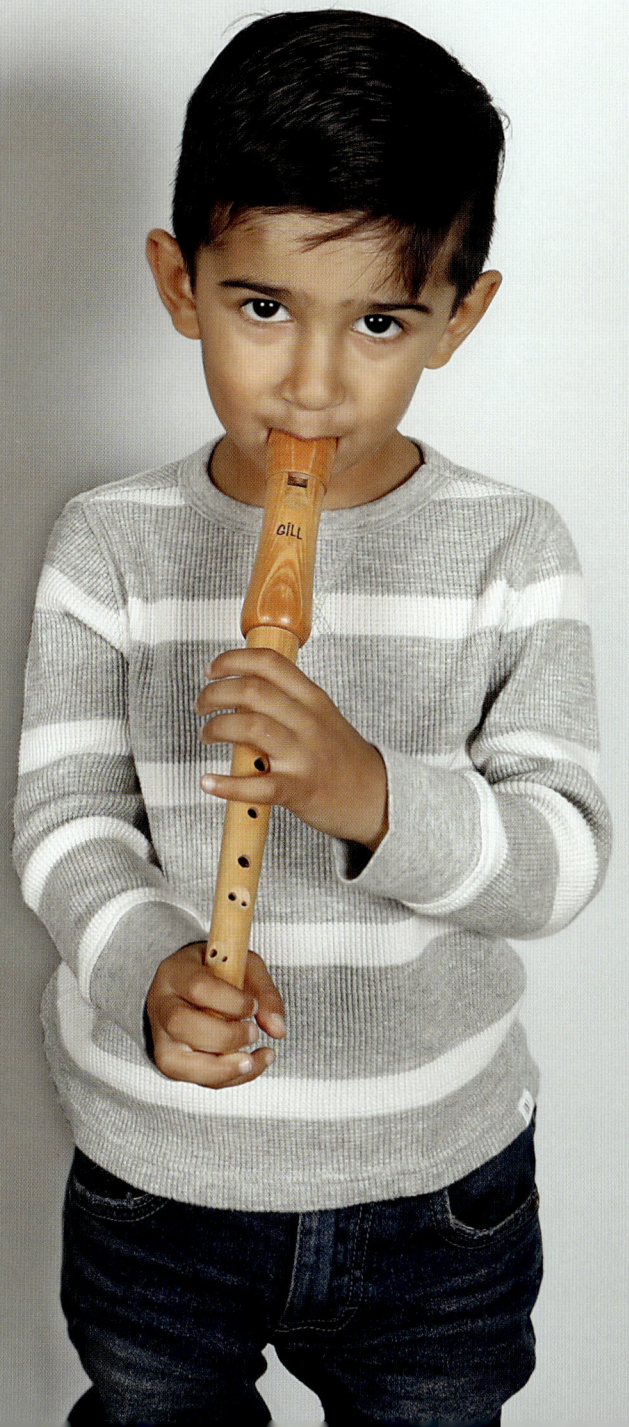

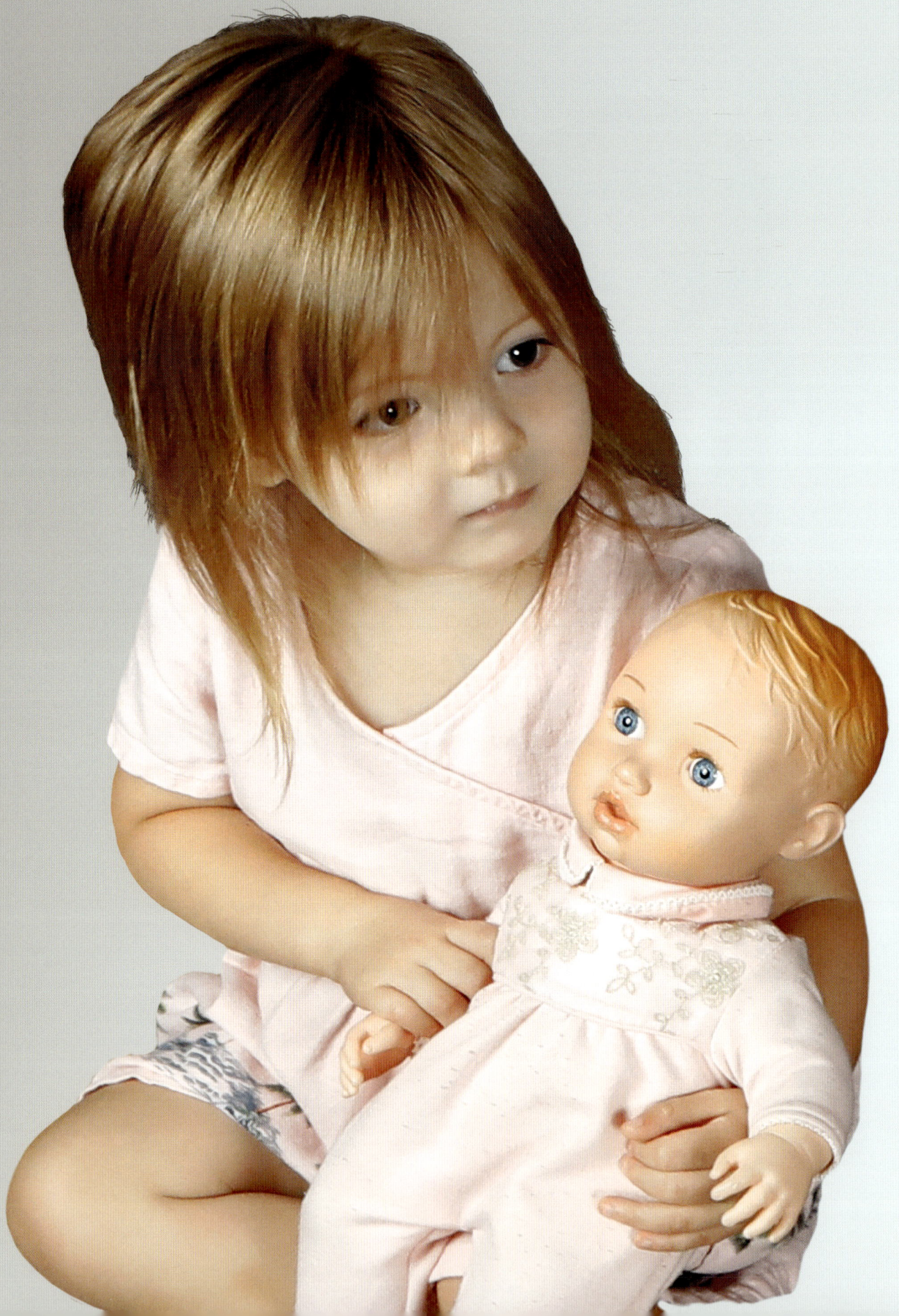

DENTAL EXAMINATION AND TIPS FOR INCREASING COMPLIANCE

This chapter explores the basics of performing a dental examination on infants, toddlers, and children. Treating infants (up to 12 months) especially can be something of a novelty, so this chapter provides advice on positioning these patients as well as lengthening children's attention spans and increasing their compliance.

First, the patient and their guardian should be afforded a short period of time to orient themselves in the waiting room. Gloves, mirrors, and a child's toothbrush should be laid out ready in the treatment room. There are differing opinions on the subject of gloves; particularly with young children (ages 2 to 3 years), many dentists recommend not using objects such as gowns, masks, or gloves on first contact, as they might be perceived as threatening.[1] Having said that, it is important to remember that even the smell of freshly disinfected hands can seem very threatening and unpleasant.

It may be helpful to use scented sprays to mask some of the smells associated with dental treatment (ie, disinfectant, latex, etc). The use of colored gloves or even wearing a different-colored glove on each hand can make a big difference in the eyes of a child. To add even more whimsy, at the end of the appointment you can turn the gloves inside out, blow them up, draw a face on them, and give them to the child. Pediatric dentistry should be all about fun.

> "We can't form our children on our own concepts."
>
> JOHANN WOLFGANG VON GOETHE

CONSIDERATIONS PRIOR TO EXAMINATION

Forms

When treating children, it is a good idea to prepare special history-taking forms or amend existing ones appropriately (Fig 4-1). A detailed history with regard to nursing, drinking, eating, and brushing habits makes it easier to prioritize, serves as a guide for the subsequent advisory discussion, and in the process uncovers many dietary traps. As with adults, it is essential

Dear Parents,

This registration form will help ensure your child's health and safety. Please read through the form and fill it out carefully. The information you provide is subject to medical confidentiality, and its sole purpose is to enable us to tailor the treatment to your child's state of health.

Family name: _____   First name: _____
Date of birth: _____
Phone number: _____
Insurance carrier and number: _____
Attending pediatrician/general practitioner: _____
Address: _____

Would you consider your child more relaxed or anxious? ☐ Relaxed   ☐ Anxious
When was your child's last visit to the dentist? _____
Has your child ever had an accident in the mouth/jaw area? ☐ Yes   ☐ No
If yes, what? _____
What is the reason for your visit to the dentist today? What concerns do you have?
_____

Stage of development
Was your child born to term? _____
Has your child taken medication frequently? _____
Does your child have siblings? ☐ Yes   ☐ No
If yes, how many? _____ What are their age(s)? _____
At what age did your child get their first tooth? _____

State of health
Has your child had or does your child have a disease of the heart? ☐ Yes   ☐ No
Check any that apply:
☐ Congenital or acquired heart defect
☐ Heart surgery
☐ Other _____

Are immunizations up-to-date? ☐ Yes   ☐ No
Does your child have any of the following illnesses?
☐ Blood disease   ☐ Infectious disease (HIV, hepatitis, TB, etc)
☐ Clotting disorder   ☐ Hearing difficulty
☐ Diabetes   ☐ Poor eyesight
☐ Respiratory disease   ☐ ADHD
☐ Rheumatic disease   ☐ Prone to accidents
☐ Liver disease   ☐ Skin disease
☐ Convulsions (epilepsy, etc)   ☐ Kidney disease
☐ Gastrointestinal disease   ☐ Allergies (if so, which) _____

Does your child take any medication? ☐ Yes   ☐ No
Which: _____ Reason: _____
Does your child breathe through the mouth, suck on something regularly, or have habits like grinding the teeth, chewing on a pencil, etc? ☐ Yes   ☐ No

(cont)

Fig 4-1 Example of a history-taking form for children.

Dental care

Who brushes the child's teeth?
☐ The child
☐ The parents
☐ The child with help of the parents

What is used to clean the child's teeth?
☐ Manual toothbrush
☐ Electric toothbrush
☐ Dental floss
☐ Other

When are the teeth brushed?
(Check all that apply.)
☐ Before breakfast
☐ After breakfast
☐ After lunch
☐ Immediately after evening meal
☐ Before going to bed

What products do you use?
☐ Children's toothpaste with fluoride
☐ Adult toothpaste with fluoride
☐ Mouthwash with fluoride
☐ Fluoridated water
☐ Fluoride supplements

Diet

For how long was your child breastfed? _____
For how long was your child bottle-fed? _____
Does your child still drink from the bottle? ☐ Yes   ☐ No
If yes, what? _____
What does your child drink between meals?
☐ Water ☐ Milk ☐ Juice ☐ Soda ☐ Nothing ☐ Other
On a typical day, what does your child eat for the following:
Breakfast _____
Lunch _____
Dinner _____
What does your child eat in between meals? _____
Does your child regularly use sugar-free chewing-gum? ☐ Yes   ☐ No

_____   _____
Date   Signature of child's guardian

to be informed about any prior fluoride history, current medications the patient may be taking, and any allergies or systemic diseases; contact information for the patient's pediatrician should also be recorded. Patient history forms should be regularly updated. The American Academy of Pediatric Dentistry has forms like this available for download.[2]

In addition, it may be advisable to hand to parents a few useful tips for them to read in the waiting room (see Fig 2-1).

Consent

A crucial point in the treatment of children is the consent to treatment of minors. Each state has its own laws governing age of consent, so dentists must consult their state boards for complete information on this topic.

ASKING PERMISSION

It is always wise to ask the parent for permission before examining the child. This gives the parent the control they want and you the approval to proceed. This especially applies when taking radiographs; be sure to be specific about which type of radiograph you are taking and why. Some people simply love to complain, so it is best not to give them any reason to question the treatment performed by asking permission first and explaining your reasoning second.

Doctor-patient confidentiality

Again, because each state has its own laws governing age of consent, doctor-patient confidentiality may or may not apply based on the individual circumstance. Dentists should consult their state boards to determine the boundaries set for the state in which they practice.

Child abuse

If child maltreatment or abuse is suspected, the practitioner should take appropriate action according to the guidelines established by each state's department of social services. Dental practitioners should become suspicious in the following circumstances:

- The clinical findings do not fit the reported circumstances of the accident
- Signs of repeated injuries (multiple, differently colored bruises also on the contralateral side) can be identified
- If previous treatments are known to have taken place
- If a disproportionately long time has elapsed between accident and attendance at the dental practice

EXAMINING AN INFANT OR YOUNG TODDLER (UNDER 2 YEARS)

In terms of positioning an infant or young toddler, the lap examination or the knee-to-knee examination[3] has proven to be the most effective. This involves a parent adopting a comfortable sitting position and placing their child facing toward them on their lap, looking into their eyes, and holding their hands. The dentist can look down on the child from above and perform the examination (Fig 4-2). The slight overextension of the head often causes a reflex opening of the mouth, which aids the examination. There are some special lap cushions available, but even without this accessory an examination or even a treatment can be done without difficulty. The parent and the dentist should convey to the child with a wide smile and calm demeanor that this unusual situation is all right and should not be seen as threatening. A crying baby is no reason to interrupt or completely

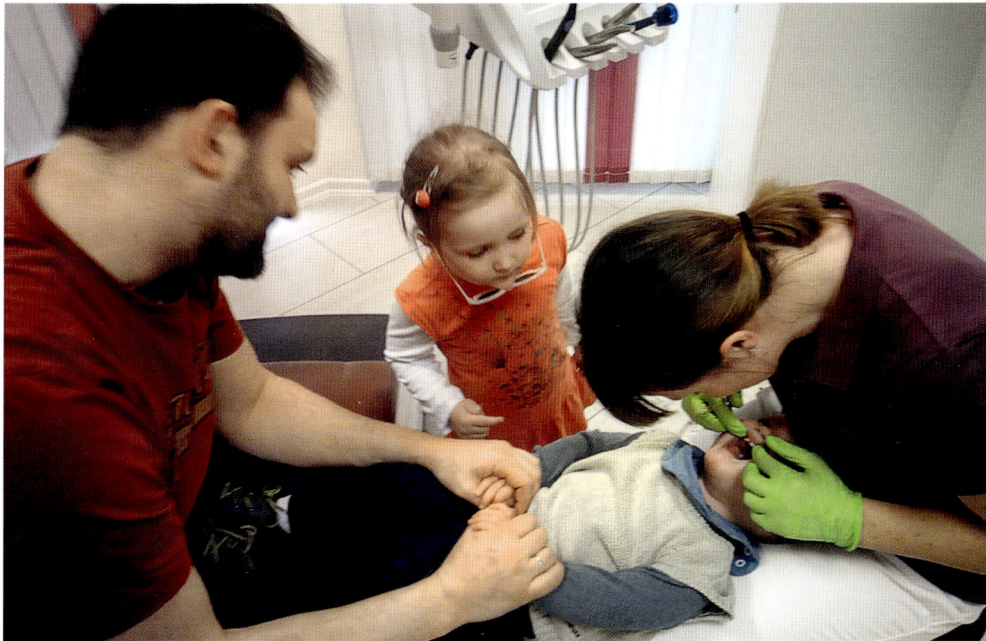

Fig 4-2 Performing a lap examination and demonstrating the lift-the-lip technique on a 16-month-old toddler.

stop the examination. The time frame has to be manageable, and these young children are generally soothed quickly in the arms of their parent.[4]

As well as any teeth that may already be present, the mucosa and frena need to be examined for any abnormalities. In addition, the child's top lip should be carefully lifted; this lift-the-lip technique (see Fig 4-2) can be demonstrated to the parents to aid daily oral hygiene (see chapter 3).

EXAMINING A TODDLER (2–3 YEARS)

Toddlers aged 2 to 3 years can be examined via the lap examination method or lying on the treatment chair, depending on their compliance and their size. Many children, especially curious toddlers, want to climb up onto the "up-and-down chair" themselves and are content for their parent to take a seat nearby. However, some children prefer to be examined lying on a parent. In that case, the child should slide up high enough so their head lies on the parent's shoulder and can be turned toward the dentist (Fig 4-3). If the child is positioned further down on the parent, mouth opening is limited because the child's chin is directed toward their chest, making examination difficult to perform.

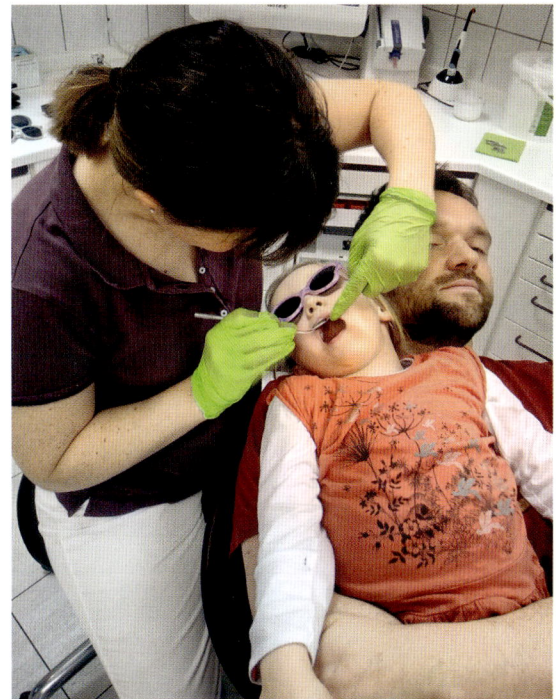

Fig 4-3 The child's head should be brought to lie on the parent's shoulder so that the dentist has good access and visibility for examination.

POSITIONING TIPS

- Most children do not like to be adjusted into a lying position in the chair and will immediately sit back up again once lowered. To prevent this, the treatment chair can be adjusted to an appropriate horizontal position before the young patient is brought into the room. In this case, most children will lie down without any problems.
- Special cushions can be used to ensure that the child is comfortably positioned if needed.
- Particularly when adjusting the treatment chair into a lying position, bodily contact with the child should be maintained (hand on the stomach, shoulder, or temples).
- Another proven method is to allow children to choose from a small selection of sunglasses to wear during the examination. Most children love selecting sunglasses for themselves and will lie there more calmly if there is no light blinding them.

INCREASING COMPLIANCE IN CHILDREN

A child is not a little adult. Children have their own emotions, perceptions, and very real fears. Therefore, a diffident child should not be spoken to loudly or put under pressure. Instead the dentist should try to allay any fears. Instead of unfamiliar dental materials, familiar things such as their own toothbrush can be used for the examination. Sometimes it can help to let children clean their teeth first and then give them praise. The self-confidence gained may increase patient compliance. Other children find it calming for a parent or a sibling to hold the dental mirror.

Stuffed animals can sometimes help children overcome boundaries and allow dental staff to intrude on the intimate area of the mouth. A lot of children are able to venture beyond their boundaries if a more experienced sibling is examined first and then praised. Furthermore, the previously described method of reflecting behavior with a hand puppet can help to remove fear of contact (see chapter 2). It can also help to create trust if young patients examine their favorite stuffed animal themselves or the dentist does so.

It is important to remember that children have a much shorter attention span than adults. In fact, an attention span of about 5 minutes per year of life is to be expected.[5] Because of this, it can be helpful to stimulate children's curiosity and keep them engaged during the examination. Asking questions like "Do you have little boy's teeth or little girl's teeth?" and "How many teeth do you think you have in there?" invite the child into the conversation and generally segue into counting the teeth, which most children enjoy.

The aim is always to complete the examination with a positive outcome. Even if a visit has only gone moderately well, the dentist should pick out something that can be praised ("Today you let me peek into your mouth to see how well your mommy cleans your teeth. Next time I'd like to be able to count your teeth."). A small prize before leaving is always popular. Oftentimes the promise of a prize is enough for even the shyest children to at least open their mouth for the briefest of moments. However, if the child outright refuses to be examined, he or she should not be rewarded with such a prize. This is uncommon, and nevertheless the dentist should always strive to find something positive to praise the child for.

Furthermore, the entire team can contribute to increasing overall compliance by integrating children into the practice in fun ways. For example, a bell can be kept in an easily accessible place in the office, and the staff can ring it as a sign of praise for a child doing something good or the child can even ring it themselves if possible. Kids love to be included in their treatment and made to be feel special like this. Another idea is to host a coloring contest to engage the kids and using the winner's art for marketing purposes. The more you can engage your pediatric patients, the better chance you have of them feeling comfortable, being compliant, and most importantly, being motivated for good oral health.

IT'S ALL ABOUT FUN!

The more fun a kid has in your office, the more compliant he or she will be. Make sure you have fun toys, you hand out cool prizes, and you engage the child in fun ways.

IMPORTANCE OF TAKING NOTES

It is very helpful to take notes after the examination in order to tailor your approach to the follow-up appointment based on the child's initial compliance. The following should be noted: how the child participated, whether he or she sat alone in the chair, whether the child willingly showed his or her teeth, whether the child was anxious, and what arrangements were made for the next appointment. This simplifies the next appointment because it can be linked to the previous one, not to mention that it creates a familiar atmosphere where the child feels important and remembered by the dentist.

REFERENCES

1. Zehner G. Quick Time Trance und Hypnopunktur. http://www.kinderzahnarzt-praxis.info/app/download/5872895961/QuickTimeTrance+- und+Hypnopunktur.pdf?t=1359880533. Accessed 2 December 2016.

2. American Academy of Pediatric Dentistry. Medical History Form. https://www.aapd.org/globalassets/media/policies_guidelines/r_medhistoryform.pdf. Accessed 4 February 2020.

3. Viswanathan K. Infant oral exam and first dental home. Tex Dent J 2010;127:1195–1205.

4. Beck J, Eßer W, Gösling J, et al. Praktischer Ratgeber für die zahnärztliche Praxis. Frühkindliche Karies vermeiden. http://www.kzbv.de/ecc-ratgeber-einzelseiten-2016.download.78b1eb79e732ea8b84fb-d65a60ccbc60.pdf. Accessed 2 July 2016.

5. Atzlinger F. Kinderhypnose in der Zahnheilkunde [thesis]. Universität Budapest, Fakultät für Zahnmedizin, 2008. http://www.zahn1.at/service/downloads?file=files/assets/content/Download/DiplomarbeitKinderhypnoseinderZahnmedizinges.pdf. Accessed 26 August 2017.

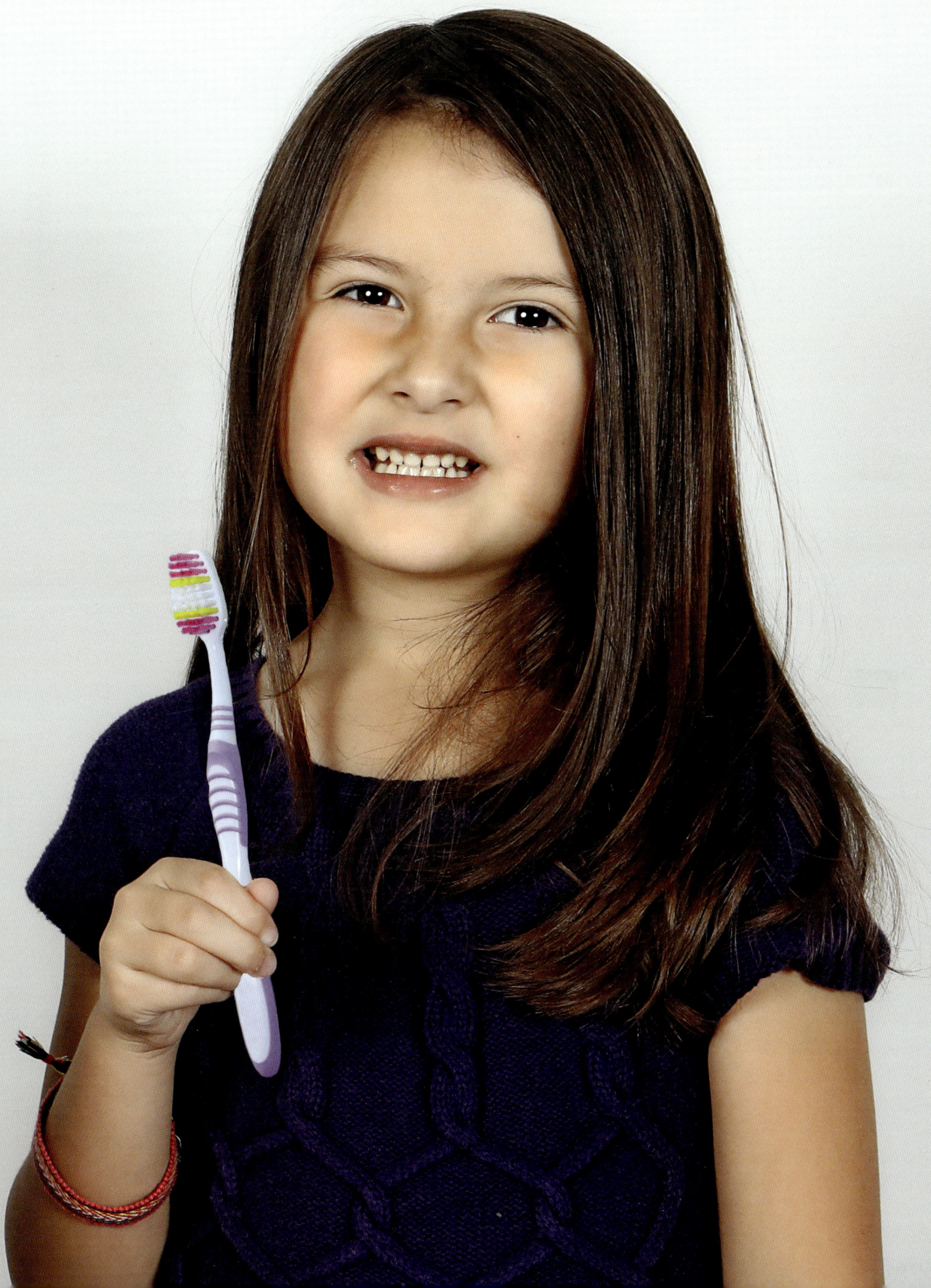

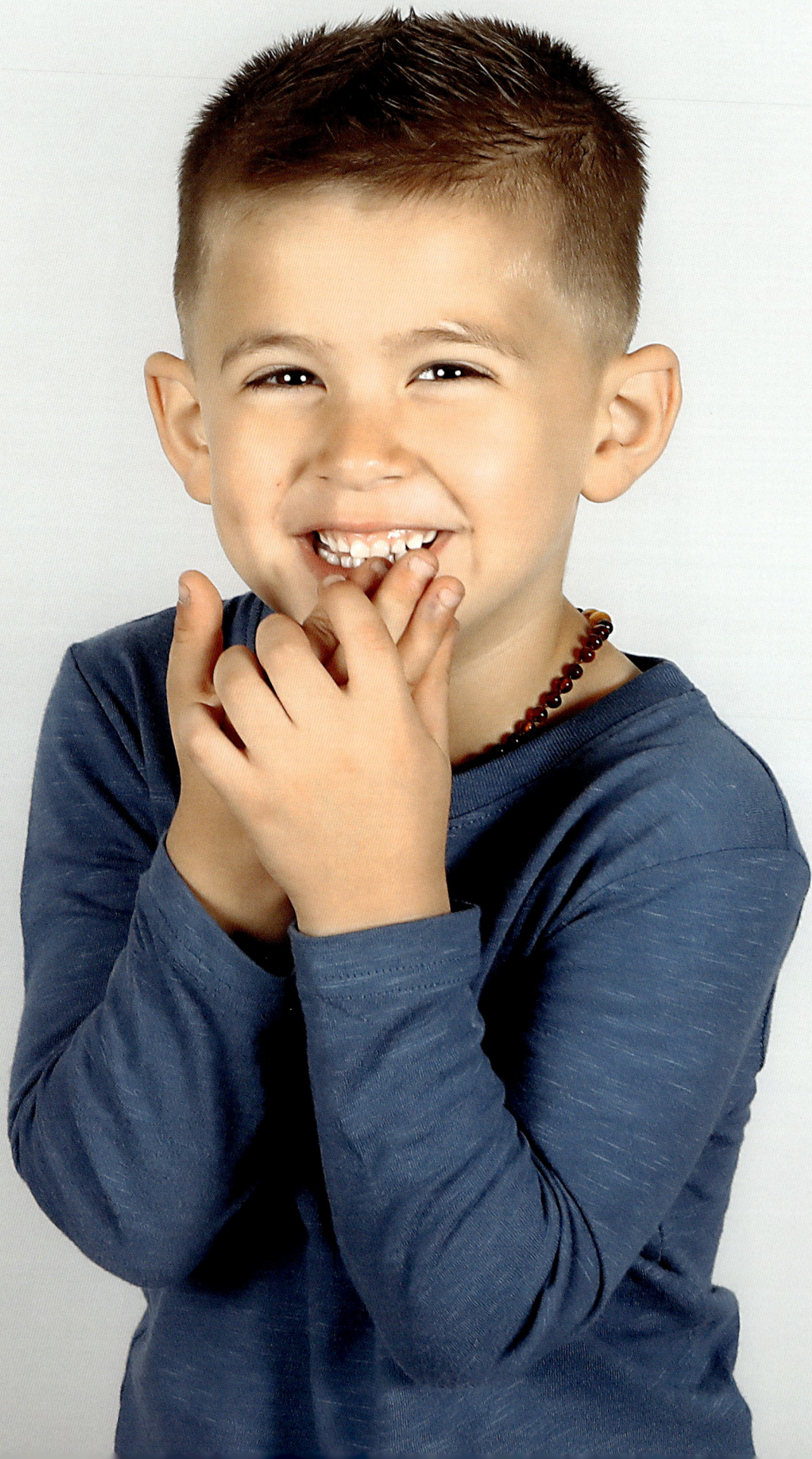

5

DIAGNOSTICS IN PEDIATRIC DENTISTRY

Dental diagnostics in pediatric dentistry is essentially no different from that in adult dentistry. During the course of the dental checkup, all the teeth, the position of the teeth and jaws, and the mucosa and soft tissues are assessed. Especially with children who are constantly going through a dynamic process of development and growth, it is important to not focus solely on the mouth. This chapter pays particular attention to myofunctional diagnostics because *(1)* children often have habits that can adversely affect the muscular balance in the maxillofacial area, which plays a major role in the healthy development of teeth and jaws, and *(2)* myofunctional diagnosis and treatment is still uncharted territory for many dentists. In addition, radiodiagnostics are covered to remove uncertainty regarding the appropriate use of radiography in children.

"First the observations and then the experiment, then thinking without authority, testing without prejudice."

DR RUDOLF VIRCHOW

"I SPY WITH MY LITTLE EYE"

Most general dentists use light, air, and a magnifying loupe for basic diagnostics. However, it is difficult to diagnose approximal caries because many children already have no gaps in their primary dentition and tight interproximal contacts, and caries will not become visible on radiographs until there is mineral loss of at least 10% to 20%.[1] Studies show that, even in social strata with a low risk of caries, a third of 5-year-olds have approximal lesions that were undetectable on visual examination (Fig 5-1). Of course, there are some tools such as fiber-optic transillumination (FOTI) or laser-induced fluorescence (eg, DIAGNOdent, KaVo), which can be a great diagnostic help, but they tend not to be available in general dental practices. Therefore, it is all the more important to make full use of the aids that are available.

Furthermore, it is important to know that most caries lesions in the primary dentition are found in the interdental space between the first and second primary molars. The distal area of the maxillary primary first molar is a particularly common site for caries. The use of light and very thorough

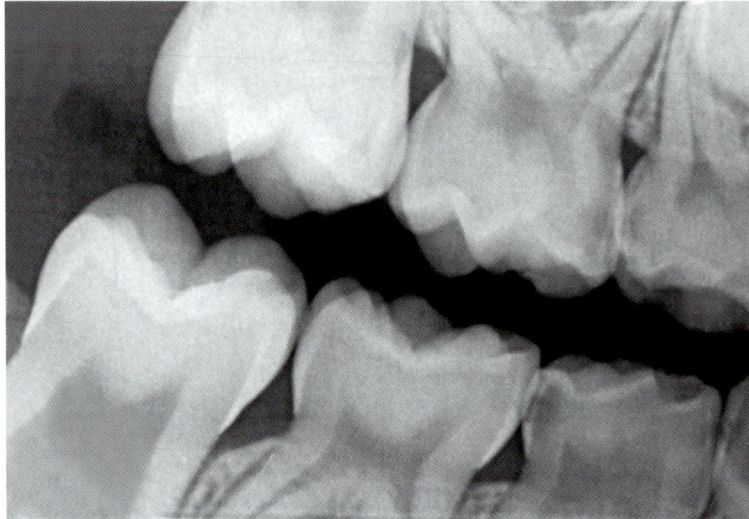

Fig 5-1 Bitewing radiograph of a 5-year-old girl (early teether) with a completely unremarkable intraoral examination. However, the lesions in the interdental space are clearly discernible.

drying of the teeth can in some cases reveal white, opaque areas. In this case, it is reasonable to assume that there is a lesion in the interdental space that is already advanced. Dental floss can also be used as a diagnostic tool; if the floss gets stuck or frays or there are food remnants in an otherwise tight interdental space, it may be evidence of caries. As with adults, the pointed dental probe is not suitable for diagnostic purposes because in some circumstances it can destroy the intact enamel surface of initial lesions.[1] If required, it can be replaced by a rounded probe. Diagnosis should always be guided by patient history and key data. For example, if a high risk of caries is likely based on patient history or previous restorative work, the dentist should quickly progress to further diagnostic measures such as radiographs.

RADIODIAGNOSTICS

Children can often talk about very diffuse, vague pains. If a child presents with such complaints, a dental radiograph of the region in question should be taken whenever possible and reasonable.

According to the guidelines of the American Association for Pediatric Dentistry, bitewing radiographs can be taken if there is evidence of disease or close proximal contact in children even prior to the eruption of their first permanent tooth. The timing of radiographs should not be dependent on the age of the patient but on the individual circumstances (Table 5-1).[2] However, as a general rule, the younger the patient, the faster one can assume the caries will progress, so history of previous caries is particularly relevant when considering radiography in young children.

TABLE 5-1 Recommendations for prescribing dental radiographs

Type of encounter	Patient age and dental developmental stage		
	Child with primary dentition (prior to eruption of first permanent tooth)	**Child with transitional dentition** (after eruption of first permanent tooth)	**Adolescent with permanent dentition** (prior to eruption of third molars)
New patient* being evaluated for oral diseases	Individualized radiographic examination consisting of selected periapical/occlusal views and/or posterior bitewings if proximal surfaces cannot be visualized or probed. Patients without evidence of disease and with open proximal contacts may not require a radiographic examination at this time.	Individualized radiographic examination consisting of posterior bitewings with panoramic examination or posterior bitewings and selected periapical images.	Individualized radiographic examination consisting of posterior bitewings with panoramic examination or posterior bitewings and selected periapical images. A full-mouth intraoral radiographic examination is preferred when the patient has clinical evidence of generalized oral disease or a history of extensive dental treatment.
Recall patient* with clinical caries or at increased risk for caries**	Posterior bitewing examination at 6- to 12-month intervals if proximal surfaces cannot be examined visually or with a probe.		
Recall patient* with no clinical caries and not at increased risk for caries**	Posterior bitewing examination at 12- to 24-month intervals if proximal surfaces cannot be examined visually or with a probe.		Posterior bitewing examination at 18- to 36-month intervals.
Patient (new and recall) for monitoring of dentofacial growth and development, and/or assessment of dental/skeletal relationships	Clinical judgment as to need for and type of radiographic images for evaluation and/or monitoring of dentofacial growth and development or assessment of dental and skeletal relationships.		Clinical judgment as to need for and type of radiographic images for evaluation and/or monitoring of dentofacial growth and development or assessment of dental and skeletal relationships. Panoramic or periapical examination to assess developing third molars.
Patient with other circumstances including, but not limited to, proposed or existing implants, other dental and craniofacial pathoses, restorative/endodontic needs, treated periodontal disease, and caries remineralization	Clinical judgment as to need for and type of radiographic images for evaluation and/or monitoring of these conditions.		

*Clinical situations for which radiographs may be indicated include, but are not limited to:

Positive historical findings

- Previous periodontal or endodontic treatment
- History of pain or trauma
- Familial history of dental anomalies
- Postoperative evaluation of healing
- Remineralization monitoring
- Presence of implants, previous implant-related pathosis, or evaluation for implant placement

Positive clinical signs/symptoms

- Clinical evidence of periodontal disease
- Large or deep restorations

- Deep carious lesions
- Malposed or clinically impacted teeth
- Swelling
- Evidence of dental/facial trauma
- Mobility of teeth
- Sinus tract ("fistula")
- Clinically suspected sinus pathosis
- Growth abnormalities
- Oral involvement in known or suspected systemic disease
- Positive neurologic findings in the head and neck
- Evidence of foreign objects

- Pain and/or dysfunction of the temporomandibular joint
- Facial asymmetry
- Abutment teeth for fixed or removable partial prosthesis
- Unexplained bleeding
- Unexplained sensitivity of teeth
- Unusual eruption, spacing, or migration of teeth
- Unusual tooth morphology, calcification, or color
- Unexplained absence of teeth
- Clinical tooth erosion
- Peri-implantitis

**Factors increasing risk for caries may be assessed using the ADA Caries Risk Assessment forms (0–6 years of age and over 6 years of age).

Fig 5-2 Multiple missing tooth germs in an 11-year-old patient. In addition, massive resorption of the maxillary right central incisor (which is clinically entirely symptom-free) and the atypical position of the premolars in the mandible can be seen. This was the first panoramic radiograph ordered for this patient.

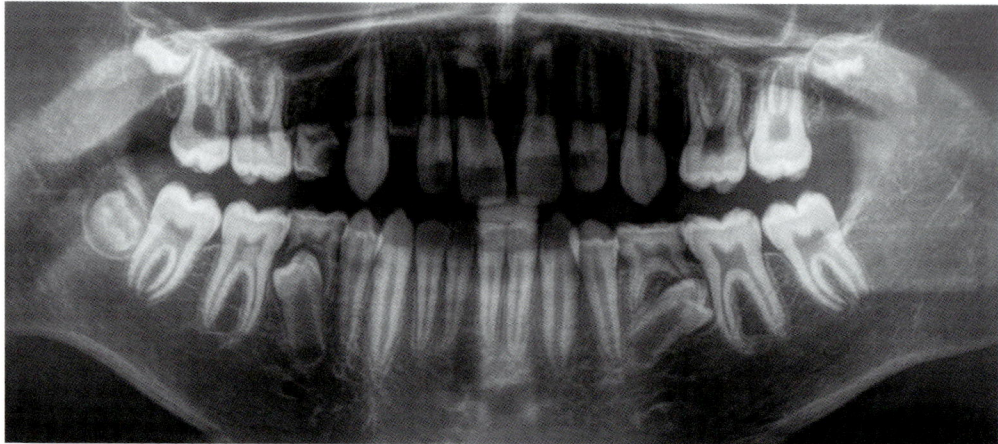

Because of the risk surrounding radiation exposure, radiographs should only be ordered when there is an expectation that the diagnostic yield will affect patient care.[2] The effects of radiation exposure accumulate over time, so good radiologic practices must be followed to minimize this exposure as much as possible. These include proper use and maintenance of the machine itself, proper film exposure and processing techniques, use of protective aprons and thyroid collars, and limiting the number of images required to obtain essential diagnostic information. According to Ermler,[1] the average annual radiation exposure from medical imaging is only 2 millisieverts (mSv) per person, which is less than the average natural environmental exposure (2.4 mSv per person), and digital techniques can further minimize this radiation exposure. Nevertheless, parents' fears should be taken seriously and addressed in a matter-of-fact discussion.

Furthermore, according to the guidelines of the European Academy of Pediatric Dentistry, bitewing radiographs should first be taken when children are aged 5 years.[3] On the one hand, they can detect approximal lesions (see Fig 5-1), and on the other hand, they sometimes reveal undermining resorption—mainly of the maxillary primary second molars—which might still be preventable in a timely fashion. Too often small carious sites go undetected in straightforward dental examinations, and 3 months later the parents come along indignant at a lesion that has collapsed. In cases with crowding of the primary dentition, the author orders bitewing radiographs even on 4-year-old children.

At times it may be necessary to perform a panoramic radiograph even in the first phase of the mixed dentition if children have parents or siblings with missing tooth germs, if eruption progresses atypically, or if there is visibly poor tooth positioning or alignment. The earlier obstacles to eruption or absent tooth germs (Fig 5-2) are diagnosed, the easier it is to search for suitable solutions in an interdisciplinary approach. If missing tooth germs are diagnosed, attention must be paid to the mineralization times of the permanent teeth (see chapter 1).

In the end, no matter what any guidelines say, taking a radiograph should always be a patient-centered decision. Each child is different, and depending on the individual caries risk we have to decide if and when we want to take a radiograph or not. What is good or necessary for one child does not have to be the right decision for another one.

TIP

Taking dental radiographs can often be used as an indicator of a child's compliance: If a child lets you take radiographs without any problems, there are usually no difficulties with other dental treatments. If a horizontal bitewing is not working, you can try to take it vertically. If the child is having trouble biting on the Rinn holder, try a Snap-A-Ray, because it is much easier for children to bite on a stick.

THE IMPORTANCE OF MYOFUNCTIONAL DIAGNOSIS

The number of myofunctional disorders that a pediatric dentist will encounter almost on a daily basis is constantly increasing. These disorders include habitual mouth breathing, a persistent infantile swallowing pattern, incompetent lip closure, tongue resting position on the mandibular anterior teeth, hypotonic lip and tongue musculature, uncontrolled saliva flow out of the mouth, and enlarged adenoids. Checking the myofunctional balance should therefore be part of any dental examination of a child in addition to checking the teeth and mucosa.

Myofunctional diagnostics, or examining the functioning of facial and oral muscles, is an extremely important element of the pediatric examination beyond infancy. Furtenbach et al summarizes the importance of myofunctional diagnosis as follows:

"The orofacial musculature, via its resting positions and the functions of breathing, sucking, chewing, and swallowing, gives the right growth and modeling impulses to the bony structures, hence their form. At the same time the form exerts an influence on the functioning processes: This involves an interaction of form and function."[4]

Growth, movement, muscles, teeth, jaws, respiration, speech—all of these elements are inseparably linked to each other. Myofunctional disorders have immense influence on the development of all the parameters of this system and ultimately on quality of life. Furthermore, orthodontic treatments will only achieve long-term success if the same diagnostic and therapeutic attention is paid to the muscles. In fact, tonsillectomies can be spared when the muscles are considered, because open mouth posture is a causal factor in the development of adenoids in two-thirds of children.[5]

The improper development of the jaw when the tongue is incorrectly positioned can be used to illustrate the importance of muscles in correcting jaw growth: As the strongest muscle in the mouth, the tongue is a key influencer for correct jaw growth. In the physiologic resting position of the mandible, the lips contact each other, and the tongue comes to lie on the palate. The patient breathes through his or her nose, and negative

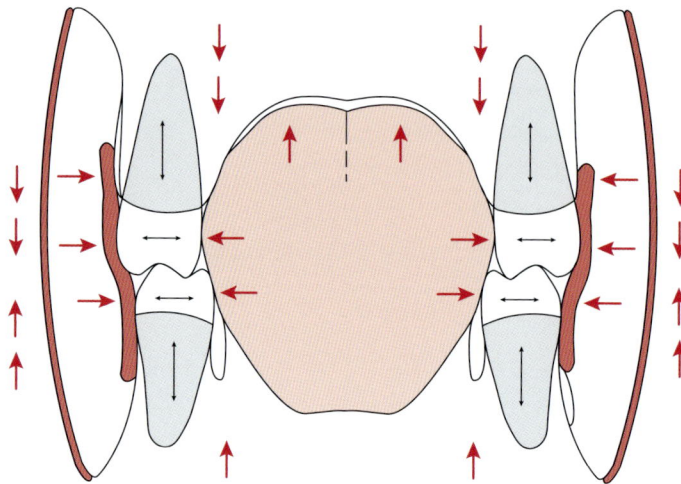

Fig 5-3 Diagram illustrating the physiologic muscle balance and its impact on the dentition in the case of competent lip closure (Courtesy of Mathilde Furtenbach.[6])

pressure prevails in the mouth. Pressure of the tongue on the palate induces proper maxillary growth and facilitates the progression of normal jaw development.

In the event of a myofunctional disorder, this cycle of negative pressure, muscle pressure, and growth induction is disrupted (Fig 5-3).[6] If the upper airways are displaced, for instance, and the child breathes through the mouth, the tongue adopts a nonphysiologic resting position in the mandible and not against the palate. As a result, growth of the maxilla is not adequately stimulated, and the mandible grows disproportionately. The consequences are occlusal anomalies, such as the development of a crossbite.[5] Competent lip closure has a huge significance in the physiologic development of the hard and soft tissues involved.

The problem with such diagnostic findings is that a vicious cycle is set up: Children who constantly breathe through their mouth suffer from respiratory diseases more often because the air they breathe in is neither warmed nor filtered.[7] As a result of frequent infections, tonsils become chronically inflamed and enlarged, which in turn makes nasal breathing difficult and can lead to middle ear involvement with conductive deafness.[5] The habitual mouth breathing in turn prevents lip closure, which causes hypotonia of the involved muscles. The risk of caries for children who breathe through their mouth increases because of the dry, poorly salivated environment; these children are also more susceptible to gingival inflammation.[7] In addition, orthodontic treatments have a higher recurrence rate.

The effects of this muscular imbalance in children are not limited to the mouth; systemic effects may also be observed. Restless sleep, snoring, digestive problems, and lack of physical resilience are just a few examples.[7] Concurrent symptoms of attention deficit hyperactivity disorder can also be observed and result in diagnostic misjudgments. In children, the only treatment is often removal of adenoids, but the problem of habitual mouth breathing and nocturnal snoring remains, which, if untreated, can cause serious sleep disturbances into adulthood.[5,8]

Grabowski subdivided the myofunctional disorders into static, passive, and active/ dynamic dysfunctions, the latter being the more aggressive disorders.[4] The following are examples of such disturbances of the muscular balance: open mouth breathing, incompetent or lack of lip closure, habitual mouth breathing, faulty swallowing pattern, or even habits such as thumb sucking.

While dentists do not have to carry out speech therapy or myofunctional therapy themselves, it is very important to diagnose myofunctional problems early in order to provide the child with the appropriate treatment as soon as possible. Children with myofunctional disorders need to be treated in an interdisciplinary way; a dentist, ENT (ear, nose, and throat) specialist, orthodontist, and speech therapist or myofunctional therapist must collaborate closely in order to ensure proper care.

Alongside dental treatment and before or during any orthodontic or ENT treatment, the young patient must undergo myofunctional therapy with a specially trained speech therapist or specific myofunctional therapist. This will strengthen the perioral and oral musculature, train the patient in nasal breathing and mouth closure, heighten awareness of correct tongue positioning, and thereby trigger all the positive side effects.[7] This patient-oriented interdisciplinary approach can avoid the need for surgical removal of the adenoids.[9] The United States is the absolute pioneer in this field and has established a specialist professional category of "oral myologist."[10] While the number of specially trained therapists is still small outside the United States, a targeted internet search for myofunctional therapists should still be performed for the patient's benefit if you practice elsewhere. Myofunctional therapy can also be used to treat habits such as thumb sucking, tongue thrusting, and so on.[7]

From what age can a child be referred for such therapy? Experience shows that it depends on the therapist and the therapeutic approach. While many myofunctional therapists start from the age of 12 months, most speech therapists feel that is too young. In such cases it may be advisable to consult by telephone before making a referral.

Tools for diagnosis

The following diagnostic features are intended to help identify children with myofunctional disorders. It should be noted that all the diagnostic characteristics listed below are only meaningful if the child is free of infection.

The initial diagnostic assessment actually starts in the waiting room as the dentist takes a focused look at the child who feels unobserved at this point. There is a probability of a myofunctional problem to be addressed if the answer "yes" is given to any of the following questions:

- While looking at the child's posture, does the general muscle tone appear rather loose?
- Is the child breathing through their mouth? Is their mouth always open?
- Is the child's tongue visible?
- Is there evidence of drooling?
- Is the child sneezing or coughing from a cold?
- Does the child look pale?
- Does the child have dark circles under the eyes? Does their face look swollen?
- Does the child have trouble hearing and appear rather absent?

In addition, indications of a myofunctional disorder can also be gathered from a patient's medical history form. Questions about any ENT conditions, type of food eaten, mouth breathing, snoring noises when sleeping, or oral habits can reveal the first indications of myofunctional disorders.

Paying close attention to things such as speech (eg, lisping), lips (eg, hypotonia), facial musculature, teeth, and jaws can eventually be used for further diagnostic assessment and can be noted on a special anamnesis form (see Fig 6-21) . Checking the swallowing pattern can also provide pointers to any disruption of the myofunctional balance. If the mentalis muscle is utilized and tensed during swallowing ("dimpled chin"), this is suggestive of a nonphysiologic movement path. Images of the relevant myofunctional findings appear in the following chapter.

Even if the subject seems complex for colleagues inexperienced in pediatric dentistry, it is essential not to let the diagnostic assessment end with the teeth and the oral mucosa. Anyone who has concerns about entering unknown territory, especially with regard to prescribing new therapies, should simply telephone their nearest speech or myofunctional therapist. Many of these colleagues offer initial diagnostic examinations of children and then establish any treatment that may be required. This type of cooperation is advantageous to young patients in so many ways, not least in terms of the prevention of caries and positional anomalies. In this context, it is also possible to consult the relevant pediatrician or an orthodontist in order to find an interdisciplinary solution.

REFERENCES

1. Ermler R. Diagnostik von Approximalkaries bei Milchmolaren mit Hilfe des DIAGNOdent pen. Berlin: Charité, Universitätsmedizin Berlin, 2009.
2. American Academy of Pediatric Dentistry. Prescribing Dental Radiographs for Infants, Children, Adolescents, and Individuals with Special Health Care Needs. https://www.aapd.org/globalassets/media/policies_guidelines/bp_radiographs.pdf. Accessed 22 January 2020.
3. Espelid I, Mejàre I, Weerjeijm K. EAPD guidelines for use of radiographs in children. Eur J Paed Dent 2003;1:40–48.
4. Furtenbach M, Adamer I, Specht-Moser B (Hrsg.). Myofunktionelle Therapie Kompakt I: Prävention. Ein Denk- und Arbeitsbuch. Wien: Praesens Verlag, 2013.
5. Grabowski R, Stahl de Castrillon F, Konrad K, Kramp B. Das adenoide Kind—ein interdisziplinäres Problem. HNO Kompakt 2010;18(3):168–174. Online verfügbar unter http://www.mft-leipzig.de/fileadmin/user_upload/Dokumente/Grabowski_Adenoide_HNO_ kompakt_3-2010.pdf. Accessed 2 July 2016.
6. Originalabbildung von Patti, Perrier d'Arc (2007); hier modifiziert von Furtenbach et al., in: Furtenbach M, Adamer I (Hrsg.). Myofunktionelle Therapie Kompakt II: Diagnostik und Therapie. Ein Denk- und Arbeitsbuch. Wien: Praesens Verlag, 2016:19.
7. Fuhlbrück S. Wie die Mundatmung Zunge, Zähne und Sprache beeinflusst. Erfahrungen mit der Myofunktionellen Therapie und der Körperorientierten Sprachtherapie k-o-s-t® nach Susanne Codoni, CH. Co-med 2010:1–5.
8. McKeown P, Macaluso M. Mouth Breathing: Physical, Mental and Emotional Consequences; Oral Health Group 2017. https://www.oralhealthgroup.com/features/mouth-breathing-physical-mental-emotional-consequences/. Accessed 14 December 2018.
9. Furtenbach M, Wallner W. Myofunktionelle Therapie (MFT) im orofazialen Bereich— praktische und kritische Aspekte aus logopädischer Sicht. (Orofacial Myofunctional Therapy—Practical and Critical Aspects from the Viewpoint of Language and Speech Therapists.) Informationen aus Orthodontie & Kieferorthopädie 2009;41:259–264.
10. Grünwald S. Myofunktionelle Therapie mit ganzheitlichen Aspekten—Eine Komplementärmethode für verschiedene medizinische Berufsgruppen; BZB; Wissenschaft und Fortbildung, 2015:64–65.

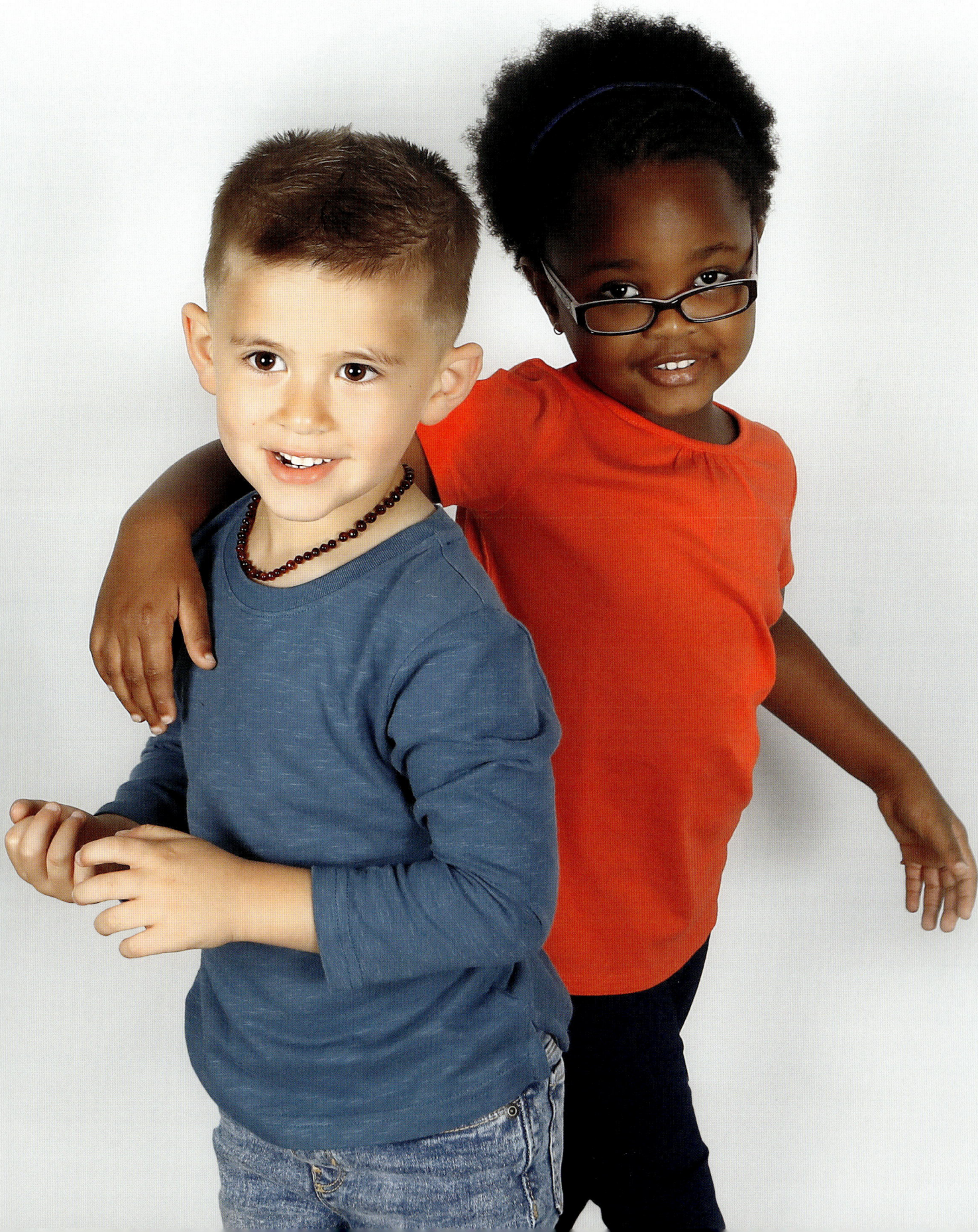

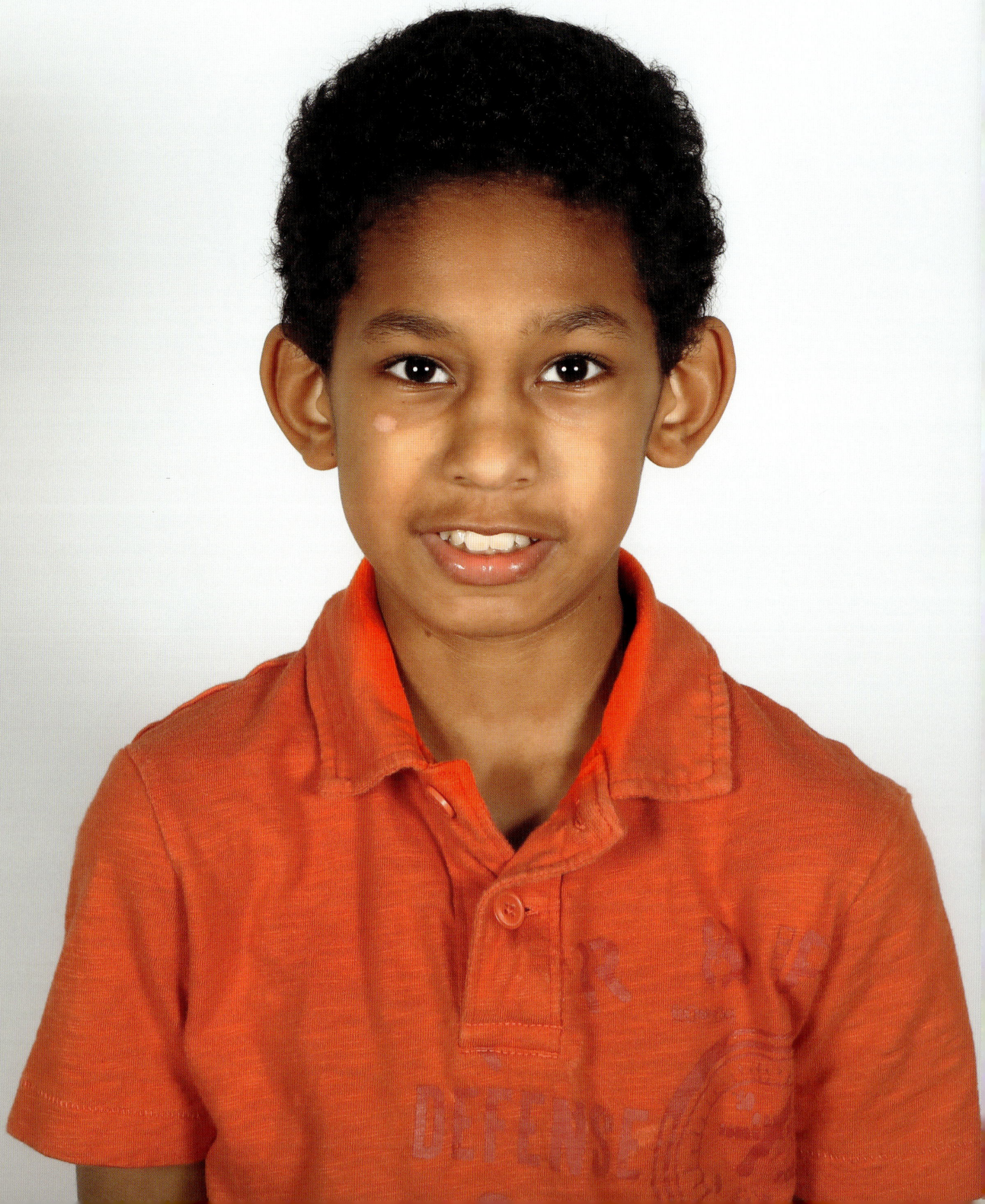

6

FINDINGS

This chapter explores various findings that are encountered commonly in pediatric dentistry. For the sake of clarity, it is divided into findings relating to the face and musculature, the oral mucosa, and the teeth, including jaw and tooth position. Diseases or syndromes that occur very rarely are beyond the scope of this chapter because they usually do not occur in a general dentistry office; in case of uncertainty, it is **always** advisable to refer the patient to a specialist as soon as possible.

"We only see what we know."

DANIEL GARLINER

FINDINGS AFFECTING THE FACE AND MUSCULATURE

Findings recorded in pediatric dentistry should not be confined to the teeth and oral mucosa. Because children are still growing, it is extremely important to identify underdevelopment or faulty development of oral, maxillomandibular, and facial muscles for successful prevention and treatment of malocclusions and malpositioning of teeth. As well as the extraoral diagnostic assessment (see chapter 5), there are some typical intraoral findings that may indicate a myofunctional disorder.

Face

Adenoid facies (or long face syndrome) denotes the typical facial morphology observed when the upper airways are narrowed due to adenoids.[1] It is characterized by an open mouth posture with a hanging lower lip; the child is usually pale, the nose looks "lifeless," and the buccal pads appear congested.[2] The child also generally appears tired and expressionless (Fig 6-1). More symptoms include disrupted lymph drainage, poor sleep, snoring while sleeping, and fatigue and lethargy during the day.[3,4]

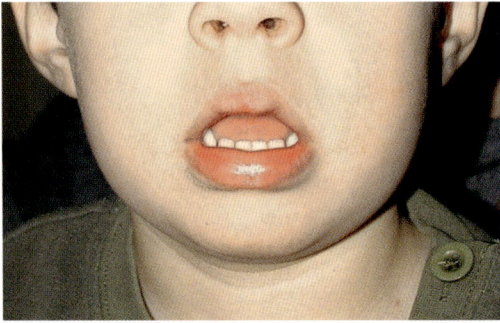

Fig 6-1 Adenoid facies. (Courtesy of Sabine Fuhlbrück.)

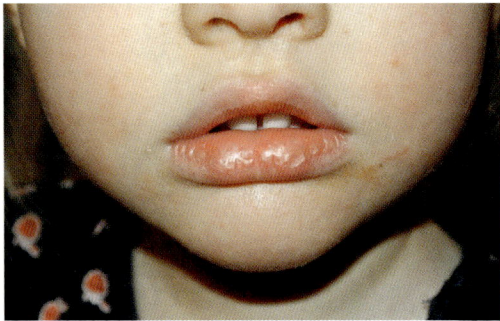

Fig 6-2 Hypotonic lip musculature and dry lips. (Courtesy of Sabine Fuhlbrück.)

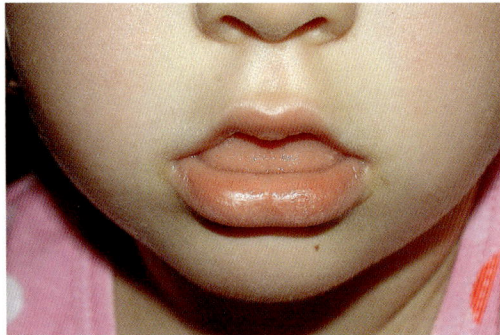

Fig 6-3 Hypotonic tongue musculature (Courtesy of Sabine Fuhlbrück.)

Nose

If a child's breathing is audible during nasal breathing while they are otherwise free of infection, this may indicate a displaced airway and an imbalance of nasal and mouth breathing.

Lips

Thick-looking lower and upper lips may be an indication of muscular hypotonia (Fig 6-2). With very thick-looking lower lips, a pronounced labiomental fold is often noticeable as well. In addition, rhagades, extremely dry or cracked lips, and tooth impressions on the lips provide evidence of oral habits.

Chin

If a child actively has to use the mentalis muscle (visible as tension in the chin area, which looks like a "dimpled chin") when asked to close his or her mouth or while swallowing, this indicates nonphysiologic compensation and disrupted muscular balance.[3]

Tongue

There may be evidence of myofunctional disorders if the tongue becomes visible when the child is swallowing. If there is an underlying nonphysiologic swallowing pattern, the tongue pushes between the teeth during swallowing and does not rest on the roof of the palate, as it normally should.[5] Impressions of teeth on the tongue may indicate oral habits such as tongue thrusting and should be investigated. A tongue that looks very large and rests on the mandibular teeth suggests muscular hypotonia and should also be investigated (Fig 6-3).

An interdisciplinary therapeutic approach is required for all these findings. If it has not yet been done by a pediatrician, the affected child should be referred to the appropriate specialist (eg, ENT [ear, nose, and throat] specialist, speech therapist, and/or myofunctional therapist), and the parents must be made aware of their child's condition.

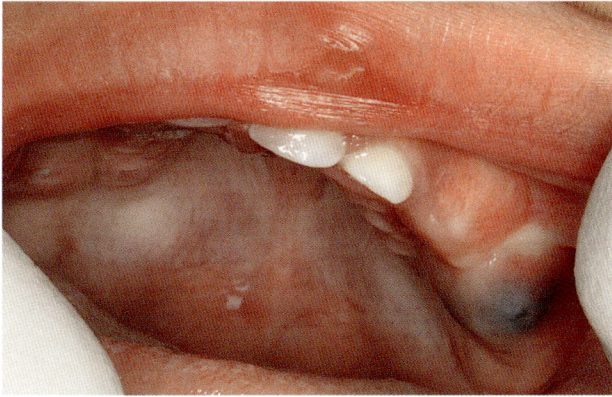

Fig 6-4 Eruption cyst in the posterior left maxilla. (Courtesy of Dr Richard Steffen.)

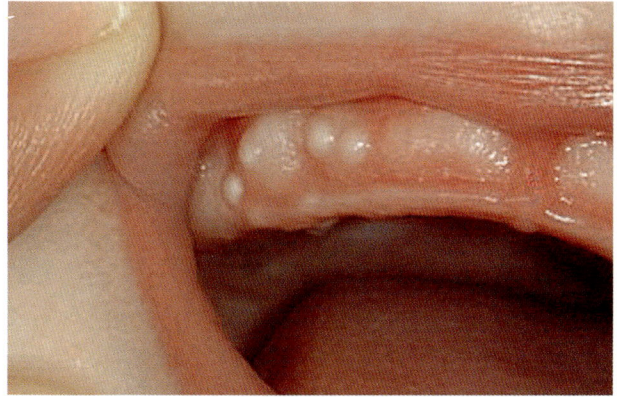

Fig 6-5 Epstein pearls. (Courtesy of Dr Richard Steffen.)

FINDINGS AFFECTING THE ORAL MUCOSA

There are some findings that appear particularly in infants and/or toddlers but are relatively rare in general dentistry practices. The list of findings included here is by no means exhaustive, and very rare clinical conditions have deliberately been omitted. In case of uncertainty regarding the diagnosis, referral should be made to a specialist and/or to a pediatrician as a matter of course.

Cysts frequently occurring in childhood

Eruption cysts
Eruption cysts are often shiny and bluish in appearance and precede eruption of the teeth (Fig 6-4). They usually do not require any separate treatment and will disappear by themselves. They often occur several times in a single child. Occasionally eruption cysts are painful for the children affected.[6]

Epstein pearls
Epstein pearls look like small white bumps on the palate or the alveolar ridge (Fig 6-5). Treatment is not necessary because the keratin-filled cysts disappear by themselves.[6]

Oral manifestations of common childhood illnesses

There are several childhood illnesses that manifest as oral efflorescences (ie, rash or lesion). The following section examines common childhood diseases only; rare conditions are not addressed. If a systemic disease is suspected, children should generally be referred to a pediatrician because it may be necessary to administer an antibiotic in certain circumstances. If uncertain lesions cannot be assigned to any systemic disease, diagnostic investigation together with an oral surgery consult is required.

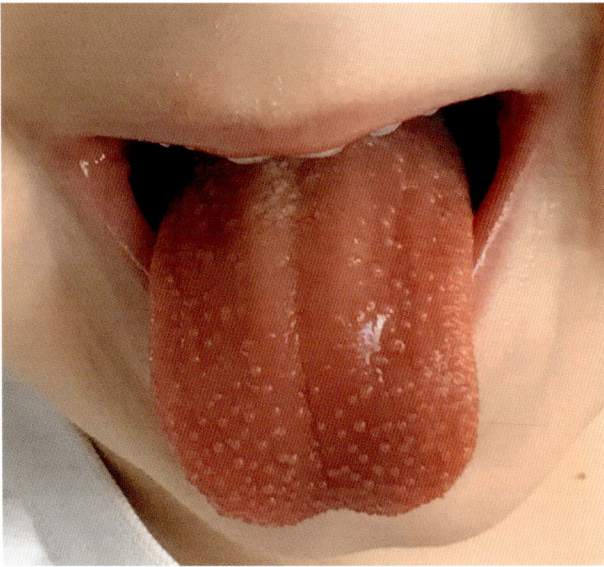

Fig 6-6 Strawberry tongue.

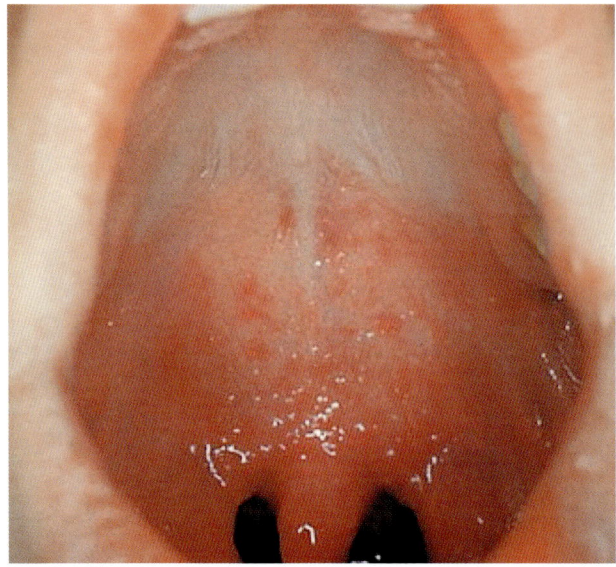

Fig 6-7 Koplik spots. (Courtesy of Dr Richard Steffen.)

Scarlet fever

Scarlet fever appears as a perioral pallor while the rest of the face is red. Other characteristic features are purulent stippling of the tonsils, reddening of the lips, and reddening of the tongue, known as "strawberry tongue"[7] (Fig 6-6).

Mumps

With mumps, bilateral swelling of the parotid glands is often noticeable, and in some cases the ear lobes may even stick out. The saliva is clear.[7]

Measles

As early symptoms of measles, the typical Koplik spots can be seen in the buccal mucosa.[7] These white spots look like grains of salt on a bright red background (Fig 6-7).

Rubella

Spotty changes to the oral mucosa of the soft palate appear as an early symptom of rubella (ie, German measles or "three-day measles").[7]

Chickenpox

Oral symptoms are bright-red, very painful, raised sores on the gingiva that often transition into ulcers. As the rash on the rest of the body is highly typical, the diagnosis is usually clear-cut in this case.

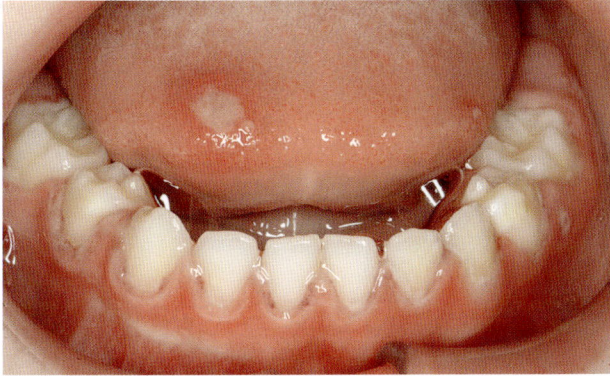

Fig 6-8 Herpetic gingivostomatitis. (Courtesy of Dr Richard Steffen.)

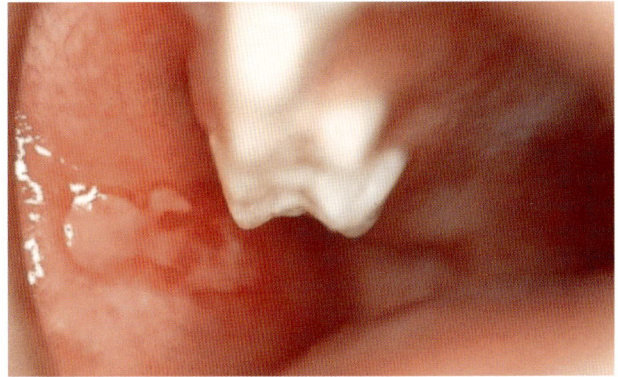

Fig 6-9 Hand, mouth, and foot disease. (Courtesy of Dr Richard Steffen.)

Herpetic gingivostomatitis (ulcerative stomatitis)

Children affected suffer from very painful blister-like lesions (Fig 6-8). The gingiva is usually swollen and bright red, and the child often gives off a typical fetid breath (halitosis). It may be difficult to eat, and oral hygiene can be severely impaired.[7] Intraoral treatment is symptomatic, involving instructions on careful oral hygiene, possibly with the use of alcohol-free chlorhexidine gluconate mouthwash (depending on age) and oral pain relievers. Caution is advisable with lidocaine or benzocaine gels because they are difficult to dose. Because of the possibility for overdose in small children, systemic pain relief with ibuprofen or acetaminophen may be safer for use at home.[8] It is important to ensure adequate fluid intake. In severe cases of herpetic gingivostomatitis, a pediatrician must be consulted.

Hand, foot, and mouth disease

Partly confluent, vesicular lesions form on the oral mucosa, mostly starting buccally, and are quick to ulcerate (Fig 6-9). The surrounding mucosa is bright red, and there are lesions on the child's hands and feet. Once again treatment is purely symptom management with analgesics.[7]

Infectious mononucleosis

As well as swollen lymph nodes, fever, fatigue, and tonsillitis, around 15% of patients exhibit numerous small petechiae on the oral mucosa, often in the area of the soft palate. Children are less commonly affected; the disease usually does not occur until adolescence.[9]

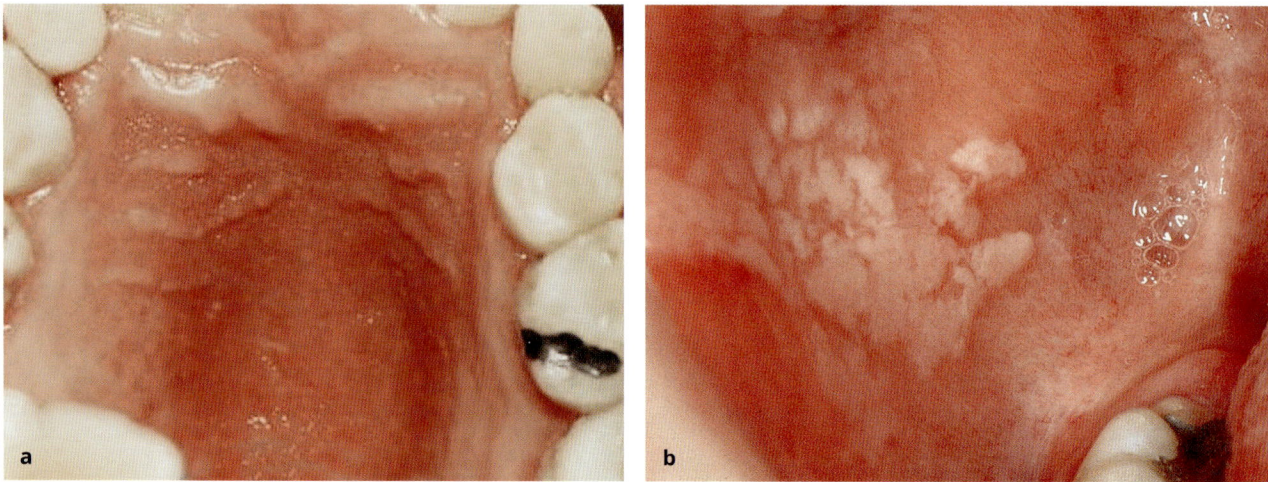

Fig 6-10 *(a)* "Sugared palate" due to candidiasis. *(b)* White mucosal change in candidiasis. (Courtesy of Dr Richard Steffen.)

Color changes to the oral mucosa

Oral thrush

Grayish-white patches on the oral mucosa that are difficult or even impossible to wipe off[10] are relatively common in infants (Fig 6-10). Unlike the whitish coating that is found in the oral cavity immediately after breastfeeding, any attempt to wipe off these white areas leaves behind small spots that bleed. The condition can be treated with nystatin or miconazole preparations, and nursing mothers should also apply the medications to the breasts. If fungal infections recur very frequently, patients should visit a physician to assess for a possibility of other underlying diseases (such as diabetes), and the infant should be checked for a tongue-tie. If a baby suffers from a tongue-tie, the mobility of the tongue is restricted; the tongue is attached to the mandible and can hardly be lifted up. Therefore, it cannot be wiped clean at the palate. This can result in a persisting white coating on the tongue or can even favor oral thrush.

Pigmented changes

Malignant pigmented changes to the oral mucosa are very rare in children. However, sharply defined pigmented changes to the gingiva that appear very suddenly are relatively common in young children; these are usually impacted food residues showing through the thin gingiva (Fig 6-11). As a result of the very loose junctional gingival epithelium, inflammation does not necessarily develop, and the course of the condition may be entirely asymptomatic, even if the foreign bodies are not removed for days. These food remnants can usually be removed without difficulty using air spray, or they will disappear by themselves within a few days.

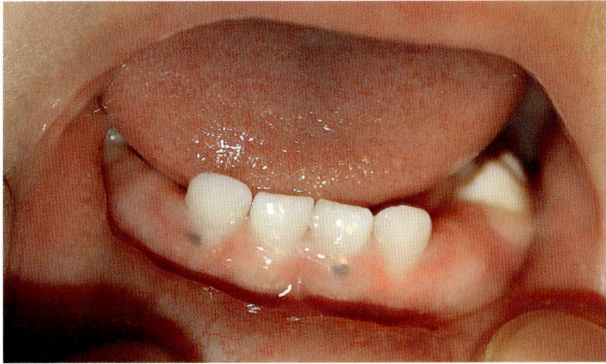

Fig 6-11 Food remnants trapped under the gingiva near the mandibular anterior teeth.

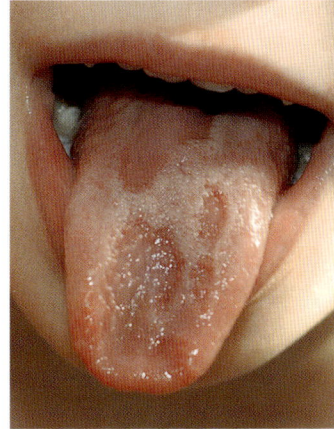

Fig 6-12 Geographic tongue. (Courtesy of Dr Richard Steffen.)

STOMATOPEDIA

The online atlas of Dr Richard Steffen provides a very good diagnostic tool. A straightforward, free registration process gives access to a wealth of image material (www.stomatopedia.com). The descriptions of the diseases and symptoms are written in English.

Changes to the tongue

Geographic tongue

This refers to typical changes to the dorsum or the margin of the tongue characterized as a white or yellowish rim with a reddened center (Fig 6-12). These areas can migrate, and a subjective burning sensation or pain is possible. Spontaneous remission can occur.[11]

Labial and lingual frena

The labial frenum and especially the lingual frenum are often neglected in clinical examinations. An added complicating factor is that there are no standardized diagnostics, and the therapeutic benefit of this diagnostic method has frequently been the subject of controversy. It is a fact that a short lingual frenum (frenulum breve or tongue-tie) in particular greatly inhibits an infant's ability to feed and can also cause the mother pain during nursing. It can also have an adverse effect on later speech development, not to mention other negative side effects such as snoring, mouth breathing, malocclusion, or extended bed-wetting if left uncorrected. Many midwives and obstetricians are aware of the importance of advising parents on consulting a dentist if they notice a short lingual frenum.

Whether a lingual frenum is too short cannot be determined by visual examination alone. It is also important to ask whether the child is feeding without any problems. If parents bring a newborn to a dental examination and describe problems with nursing, feeding, or the infant's weight gain, the lingual frenum should be examined. In older children, the mobility of the tongue can be tested by asking the child to lick the corner of the mouth or the lips or click their tongue. It should be possible for the child to bring the anterior third of the tongue up to the palate with the mouth open to an interincisal distance of at least 2 cm.[2]

If it is suspected that a lingual frenum is too short and causing functional limitations, especially with respect to pain-free, physiologic breastfeeding, excision should be performed in the infant. Older children may be prescribed myofunctional treatment/ speech therapy, or a surgical intervention will have to be carried out. A rather cautious approach to surgical intervention should be adopted with labial frena, especially in the primary dentition. Even very low-attached labial frena in infants do not necessarily impede nursing. More crucial than the morphologic characteristics of the labial frenum is the mobility of the upper lip: The infant cannot successfully feed physiologically if the upper lip cannot be turned outward because of the poor seal to the mother's breast or bottle nipple. In these very rare cases, excision of the labial frenum may be necessary, depending on the infant's age. It should be noted, however, that an excessively short lingual frenum is far more commonly the cause of nursing problems. The principle for older children is that, if the upper labial frenum extends so far that the child's phonation is impeded, excision may be indicated for speech reasons.[2]

Surgical intervention to the labial frenum due to orthodontic reasons should be postponed until eruption of the permanent lateral incisors occurs or, according to some dentists, even until the permanent canines erupt.[12] Not only is a child's compliance much better at an older age, but the indication for surgery after the "ugly duckling stage" of tooth eruption can be established with far greater certainty if it is clear whether a diastema exists, which is caused by a low-attaching labial frenum. Spontaneous space closure is still possible until exfoliation of the anterior teeth is completed. Excision should be performed with great caution: A simple incision through the labial frenum may be the right option for an infant with breastfeeding difficulties but is not sufficient or expedient when carried out for orthodontic reasons in older children. Chapter 7 provides further information about surgical intervention to the lingual and labial frena.

FINDINGS AFFECTING THE TEETH

Apart from caries of primary teeth, there are often other findings affecting the teeth in the primary dentition. Rare forms of dysplasia such as amelogenesis imperfecta are not discussed below; such complex cases should be treated by specialists.

Black stain

Black stain refers to black punctate or linear discolorations that are located in the cervical third of the tooth and adhere very strongly because this form of plaque is inclined to mineralization (Fig 6-13). The majority of studies have revealed that children with black stain have a lower risk of caries.[13] The discolorations can be removed without difficulty as part of prophylaxis, but they often reappear. Adults are only rarely affected because the stains usually disappear by themselves after puberty.[14]

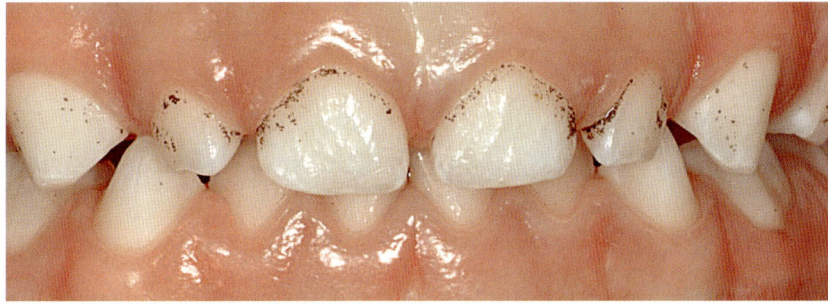

Fig 6-13 Black stain. (Courtesy of Prof Roswitha Heinrich-Weltzien.)

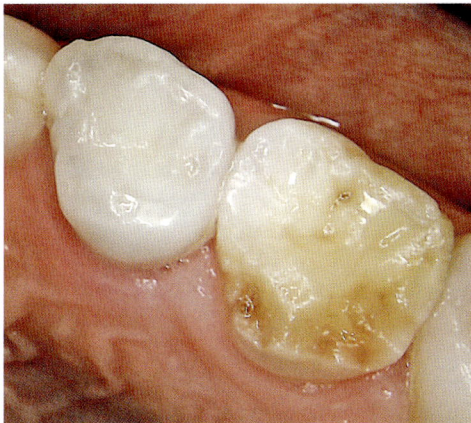

Fig 6-14 PMH affecting a primary second molar.

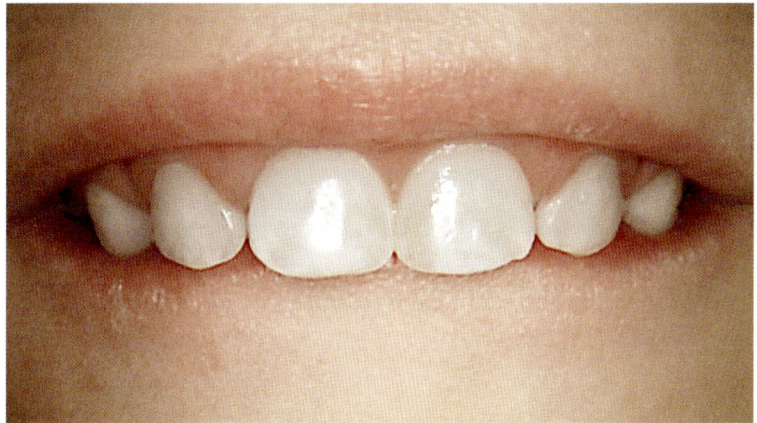

Fig 6-15 Decalcification of the primary anterior teeth in a case of habitual mal-positioning of the lower lip between the anterior teeth, causing incompetent lip closure and mouth breathing.

Hypomineralization disorders

There are two subcategories of hypomineralization disorders that are on the rise—molar-incisor hypomineralization (MIH) and primary molar hypomineralization (PMH). The prevalence of these disorders fluctuates very widely, reaching up to 21%.[15] Children who are affected by PMH have an increased risk of developing MIH and should be closely monitored in this regard.[16] The teeth appear brittle, porous, and discolored, and they abrade far more quickly (Fig 6-14). Further explanations of hypomineralization disorders and their treatment are given in chapter 7.

White spots

White spots are often the first signs of decalcification, especially on primary anterior teeth (Fig 6-15). These should not be examined with a dental probe. Instead, fluoride varnish can be applied very selectively.[17] Increased mouth breathing may be another reason for demineralization in the form of white spots. Based on the information parents gave on the medical history sheet regarding mouth breathing, drinking, eating, and oral hygiene habits, the reason(s) for these demineralizations must be determined in order to provide an individual, child-centered prophylaxis and treatment.

Fig 6-16 Discoloration of a primary incisor resulting from a previous trauma. (Courtesy of Dr Juliane von Hoyningen-Huene.)

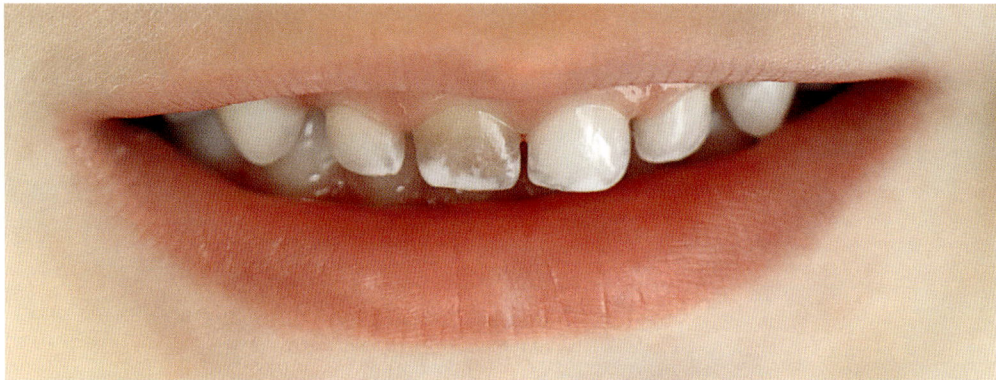

Therefore, parents should be advised on proper oral hygiene, healthy drinking and eating habits, and fluoride treatment for dental prophylaxis. High-risk patients like these should be scheduled for recall at least every 3 months, and referral to a specialist may become necessary if the lesions progress and there is a greater need for treatment.

Pink spot disease/discolorations

If a primary tooth shows increasing pink discoloration, resorption due to a prior trauma probably exists. Pink spot disease can be radiographically diagnosed; removal of the affected primary tooth is indicated in such cases. Endodontic treatments should only be considered in exceptional cases, provided that patient compliance is excellent and resorption is very limited. The resulting gap in the anterior dentition does not need to be restored from a functional standpoint.[18]

Primary anterior teeth often show grayish to brownish discoloration following trauma (Fig 6-16). Dentists can comfortably postpone treatment, provided the children do not exhibit any further symptoms. If the discoloration appears immediately after a trauma and disappears again, the formation of a hematoma was the probable cause. If discoloration occurs at a later stage following trauma, pulp necrosis or obliteration may be assumed. If the teeth then remain clinically symptom-free, it is possible to postpone any further action and merely carry out regular checkups. If pain symptoms, fistulae, or radiographic signs of periapical inflammation are apparent following trauma, the teeth must either undergo endodontic treatment or be extracted. Considering the often-limited compliance at this age and the fact that the indication for pulpectomy is age-limited, extraction should be the preferred course of action.[18] Chapter 7 discusses further details of trauma of primary and permanent teeth.

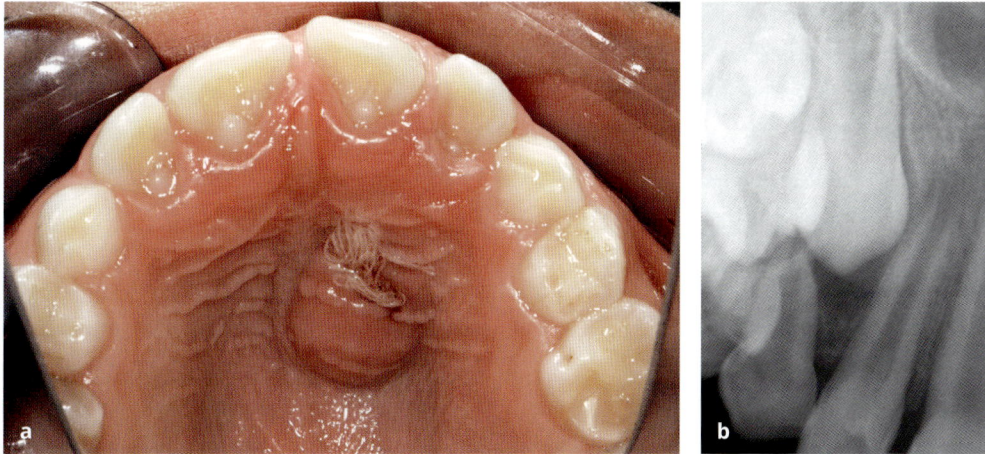

Fig 6-17 *(a)* Palatal view of a 10-year-old patient who presented with a palatal abscess with no identifiable cause. The markedly pronounced foramen cecum of the anterior teeth can be seen. The cause of the abscess was the dens invaginatus at the maxillary left lateral incisor. The drainage strips inserted can also be seen. *(b)* Radiograph of the dens invaginatus. The shadow can be seen in the region of the pulp roof. (Courtesy of Dr Gabriele Viergutz.)

A special case: Dens invaginatus

During tooth development, especially of the maxillary incisors, the foramen cecum may invaginate and cause an anomaly known as *dens invaginatus*. Depending on depth and morphology of the invagination, three different types are distinguished. In most cases, the permanent maxillary lateral incisors are affected; less commonly primary central incisors or canines are affected. The overall incidence is 2% to 7% according to the literature. In about half of affected patients, this anomaly appears bilaterally. The etiology is still not fully understood.[19]

Because these invaginations are difficult to access for carrying out oral hygiene and are not always fully covered by enamel, they are predilection sites for caries. If prompt diagnosis and prophylactic measures (eg, sealing) remain undone, the resulting untreated caries can give rise to pulp necrosis, apical periodontitis, and subsequently abscess formation (Fig 6-17a). A distinct palatal pit, abnormal coronal shapes, or slight shadows on radiographs in the area of the pulp roof (Fig 6-17b) may be an indication of dens invaginatus. Therefore, if a young patient presents with an apical radiolucency at the lateral incisor, for instance, or if this is discovered as an incidental radiographic finding without any trauma being present, dens invaginatus may be the cause. As these teeth have a particular root anatomy in some cases, referral to an endodontist is often the best option.

Malocclusion/malpositioned teeth

Crossbite

The most common occlusal anomaly in pediatric dentistry is a crossbite of individual or several teeth. If untreated, the latter can have far-reaching implications for jaw development. This is why a brief orthodontic diagnostic assessment is essential in the child's consultation.

Individual primary teeth in a crossbite position can be transposed by selective grinding. Daily spatula exercises, in which a child presses a wooden spatula to the palatal aspect of the affected teeth, can also provide a remedy. Similarly, restoration of primary teeth using a reversed primary tooth crown (lingual surface facing buccally) can effectively remedy a crossbite (Fig 6-18). Myofunctional therapy should additionally be mentioned in this context: Crossbites can be treated by strengthening the tongue muscles and reinforcing the physiologic resting tongue position or by eliminating habits that can negatively impact the mouth. If entire halves of the jaw are in crossbite, referral should be made to an orthodontist during the primary dentition phase in order to facilitate symmetric jaw growth.

Open bite

An open bite is also common. This can occur symmetrically at the midline or asymmetrically on one side. The latter has a poorer prognosis and can be caused, for instance, by sucking a thumb or finger on one particular hand only (check the child's fingers). However, an open bite may also be caused by prolonged use of a pacifier, habitual sucking on other objects (eg, blanket, stuffed animals), or a nonphysiologic tongue position/movement. It is important to eliminate the cause, if possible, and either wait to see if the bite closes or treat, depending on the child's age and the severity of the open bite. Myofunctional therapy again offers excellent treatment options. In addition, discussion with an orthodontist may of course be sought in an interdisciplinary approach.

> **TIP FOR ASSESSING JAW POSITION**
> It is sometimes difficult to get children to deliberately adopt a hinge position (maximum intercuspation), and many of them will push their mandible forward. The hinge position can help to get children to swallow, and then assess the jaw position adopted. This enables the dentist to check the swallowing pattern at the same time.

Lingual eruption of the mandibular anterior teeth

Another common finding is lingual eruption of the permanent mandibular anterior teeth where there is insufficient physiologic resorption of the roots of the corresponding primary teeth (Fig 6-19a). Parents often find this alarming, but in many cases watchful waiting will suffice. After exfoliation or, less commonly, after extraction of the primary tooth concerned, the tongue will often push the lingually erupted successional tooth into the correct position within a few weeks (Fig 6-19b).

Undermining resorption of primary molars

Undermining resorption of the primary second molar by the permanent first molar is not uncommon. If eruption of the permanent first molar is delayed on one side or they are tipped very far mesially, a radiograph should be taken for a proper diagnosis. Children

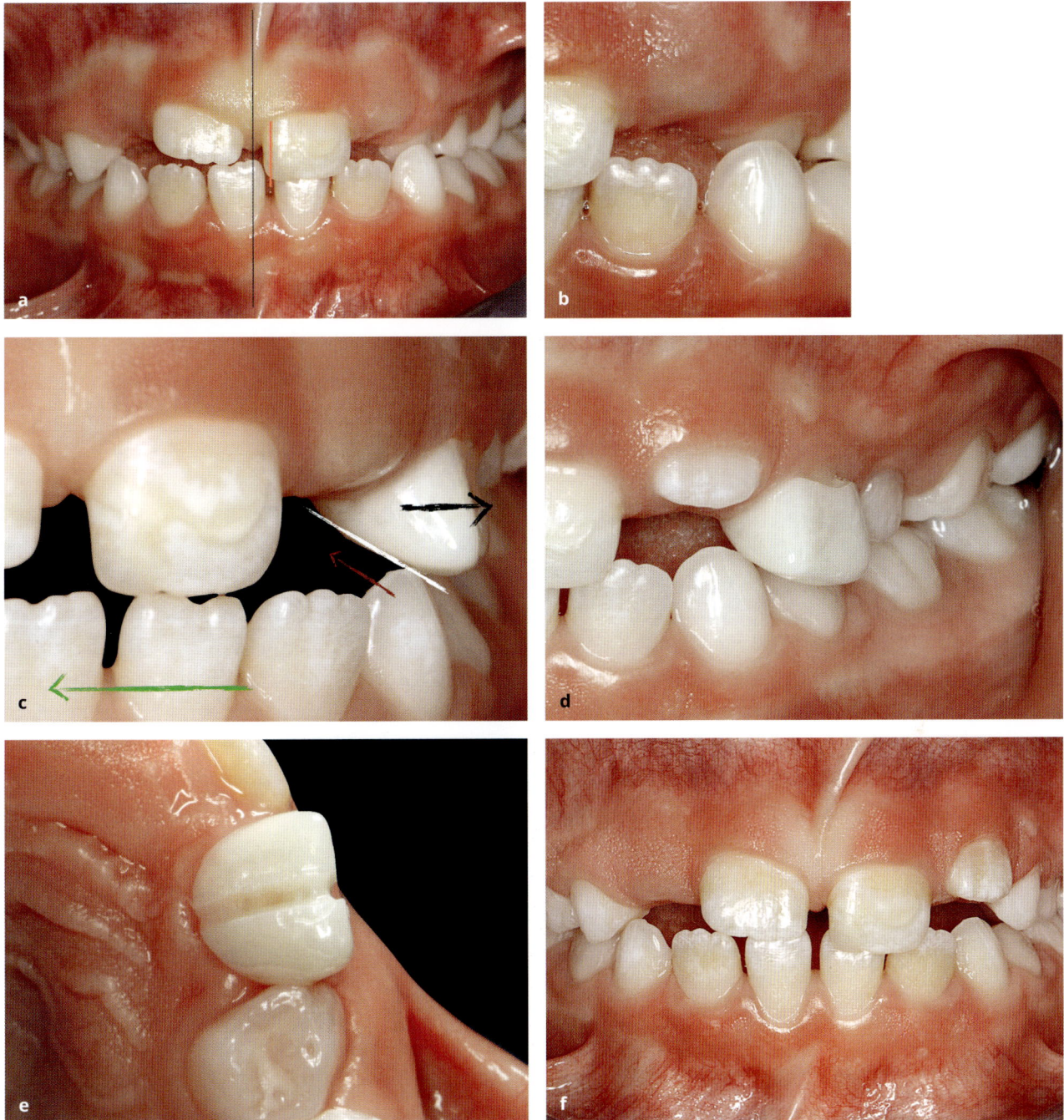

Fig 6-18 *(a and b)* The patient's midline was displaced by the crossbite in the posterior quadrants. Selective grinding measures are out of the question in this instance. *(c and d)* A pediatric crown was inserted in a reversed position (palatal side to buccal) without selective grinding of the primary tooth involved. Because of the resulting inclined plane, it was possible to correct the midline shift within 2 weeks. *(e and f)* After the desired outcome had been achieved and retained, the primary tooth crown was removed again after 8 weeks with a diamond bur under water cooling. (Courtesy of Dr Jorge Casián Adem.)

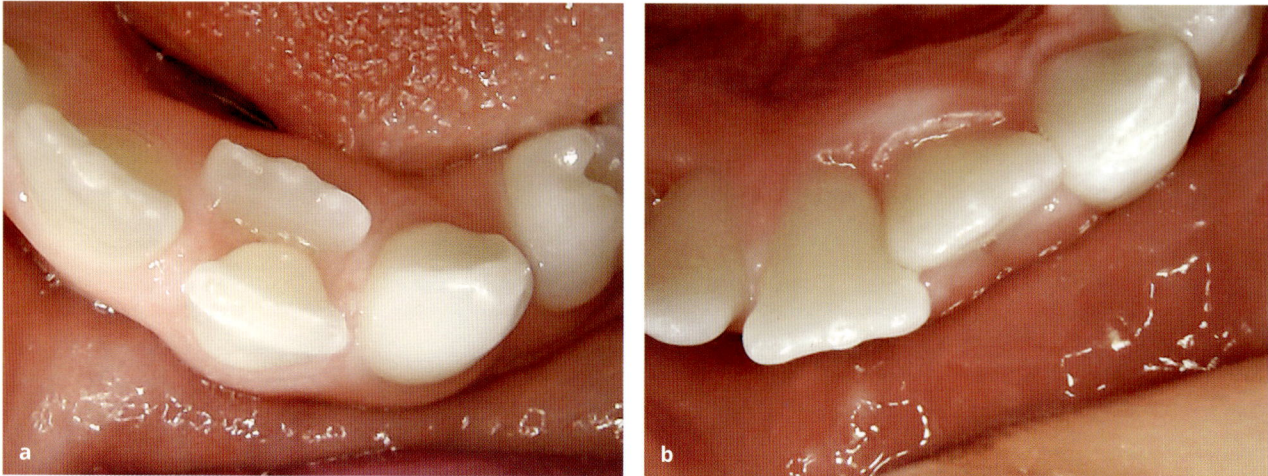

Fig 6-19 *(a)* Lingually erupting mandibular left lateral incisor. *(b)* After watchful waiting and eventual natural exfoliation of the primary tooth, the tongue pushed the tooth in the labial direction within 8 weeks.

occasionally describe pain affecting the primary second molars as well. Depending on the degree of resorption, either an attempt can be made to upright the permanent first molar in order to guarantee normal eruption (eg, using spacers in mild cases or deimpactor springs), or the affected primary first molar must be removed. In that case, space closure by the permanent first molar should absolutely be prevented. Interdisciplinary cooperation with an orthodontist is advisable.

Infraocclusion/ankylosis

Ankylosed primary molars in infraocclusion (usually the mandibular first molars) are another possibility. Ankylosed teeth should be removed; if they persist, they will impede correct jaw growth. Removal can be difficult, especially for teeth in severe infraocclusion where the distal adjacent tooth is tipped inward mesially. In these cases, it may be practical first to straighten the tipped adjacent tooth in an interdisciplinary approach with an orthodontist and only then attempt surgical extraction of the ankylosed tooth. In such cases, raising a flap and separating the primary tooth is advisable.

Resting the elevator against adjacent teeth should be avoided, especially if they are permanent teeth that have just erupted, because, in some circumstances, this can result in dislocation. Surgical removal of ankylosed primary teeth can also be referred to an oral surgeon.

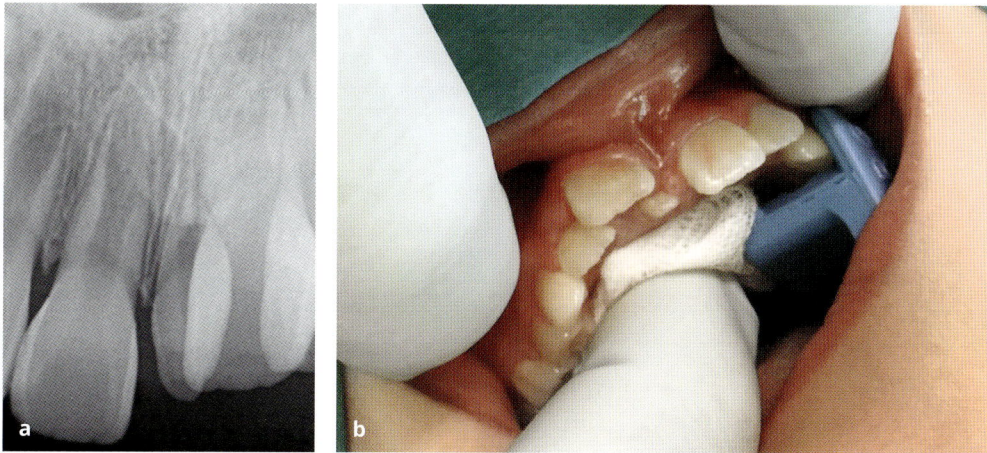

Fig 6-20 *(a and b)* Intraoral radiograph and preoperative condition of a 10-year-old patient with an already erupted mesiodens in the maxillary central incisor region. (Courtesy of Dr Matthias Nitsche.)

Delayed/atypical eruption

Atypical eruption of a permanent tooth should always give rise to further diagnostic investigation. Supernumerary tooth germs, for instance, are a possible cause. If the maxillary anterior teeth erupt entirely asymmetrically or if severely delayed exfoliation of a primary tooth occurs on one side, the presence of a mesiodens must be investigated (Fig 6-20). Intraoral radiographs or panoramic radiographs are suitable as the primary measure. If the suspicion is confirmed and appropriate removal becomes necessary, a CBCT should be performed preoperatively. By this method, any follicular cysts, root resorptions of adjacent teeth, and even the positional relationship of the teeth can be clearly diagnosed.

Further treatment is determined by a variety of limiting conditions. If the supernumerary tooth has already erupted, it should be extracted—similarly in the case of imminent or early root resorption of the adjacent teeth. If the supernumerary tooth prevents a tooth from erupting in the course of its surgical removal, the dentist should decide in an interdisciplinary consultation with an orthodontist whether a bracket should be bonded to the permanent tooth in order to align it. If the supernumerary tooth causes no problems, watchful waiting and radiographs at regular intervals (every 12 months) are indicated.[20]

CONCLUSION

Accurate and complete findings are crucial for proper treatment planning, and a good intake form can help to identify them. Figure 6-21 is an example intake form that can be used to record observations regarding the lips, tongue, cheeks, and oral habits as well as any recommendations or referrals given to the parents.

Observed Findings

Patient: _____   Dentist: _____
Age: _____
First visit on the: _____

External appearance / anomalies
Face: _____
Nose: _____
Lips: _____
Chin: _____

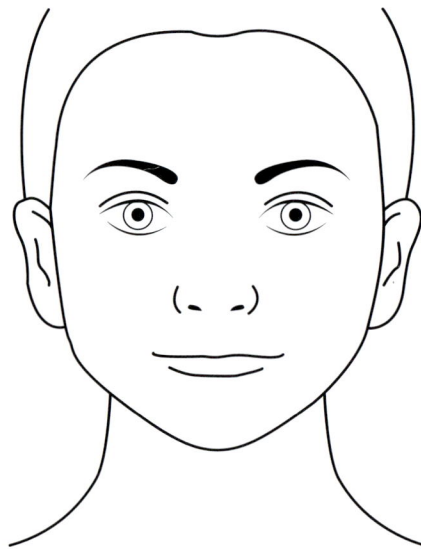

Internal appearance / anomalies
Tongue: _____
Oral mucosa: _____
Teeth: _____
Frena: _____
Orthodontic anomalies: _____
_____
_____

Function / dysfunction
Swallowing pattern: _____
Habits: _____
Breathing: _____
Tooth grinding: _____

Recommendations given to the parents / referral
_____

Fig 6-21 Intake form for observed findings.

REFERENCES

1. Grabowski R, Stahl de Castrillon F, Konrad K, Kramp B. Das adenoide Kind – ein interdisziplinäres Problem. HNO Kompakt 2010;18:168–174. http://www.mft-leipzig.de/fileadmin/user_upload/Dokumente/Grabowski_Adenoide_HNO_kompakt_3-2010.pdf. Accessed 2 July 2016.
2. Furtenbach M, Adamer I. Myofunktionelle Therapie Kompakt II: Diagnostik und Therapie. Ein Denkund Arbeitsbuch (= MFT interdisziplinär, 3). Vienna: Praesens Verlag, 2016.
3. Grünwald S. Myofunktionelle Therapie mit ganzheitlichen Aspekten. Bayrisches Zahnärzteblatt 2015:64–65.
4. Fuhlbrück S. Wie die Mundatmung Zunge, Zähne und Sprache beeinflusst. Erfahrungen mit der Myofunktionellen Therapie und der Körperorientierten Sprachtherapie k-o-s-t® nach Susanne Codoni, CH. Co med 2010:1–5.
5. Codoni S. Die Zunge im fachübergreifenden Arbeitsfeld. Hg. v. ZMK aktuell 2015. http://www.zmk-aktuell.de/fachgebiete/kinderzahnheilkunde/story/die-zunge-im-fachuebergreifenden-arbeitsfeld_1218.html. Accessed 9 December 2016.
6. Weiss P, Filippi A, Lambrecht JT. Entwicklungsbedingte odontogene Zysten. Quintessenz 2011;62:1–14.
7. Steffen R, van Waes H. Häufige Kinderkrankheiten und ihre Manifestation in der Mundhöhle. Quintessenz 2009;60:727–736.
8. US Food and Drug Administration. Risk of serious and potentially fatal blood disorder prompts FDA action on oral over-the-counter benzocaine products used for teething and mouth pain and prescription local anesthetics. www.fda.gov/ 23.05.2018. Accessed 4 June 2018.
9. Bork K, Burgdorf W, Hoede N, Young SK. Mundschleimhaut- und Lippenkrankheiten. Klinik, Diagnostik und Therapie; Atlas und Handbuch. 3. Aufl. Stuttgart: Schattauer, 2008.
10. Fuchs et al. Seltene Kinder- und Allgemeinerkrankungen und ihre Manifestation in der Mundhöhle. http://www.3d-dzb.de/media/shop/layout/home/publikation-allgemeinerkrankuungen.pdf. Accessed 4 June 2018.
11. Walter C, Sagheb K. Die Lingua geographica; zm online 2015; https://www.zm-online.de/archiv/2015/07/zahnmedizin/die-lingua-geographica/seite/alle/. Accessed 4 June 2018.
12. Clausnitzer R. Lippen- und Zungenbändchen in der Kieferorthopädie. In: Furtenbach M. Das Zungenbändchen: die interdisziplinäre Lösung. Vienna: Praesens Verlag, 2007:141–157.
13. Żyła T, Kawala B, Antoszewska-Smith J, Kawala M. Black stain and dental caries: A review of the literature. BioMed Res Int 2015:469392.
14. DGZMK: Schwarze Zahnverfärbungen bei Kindern. DGZMK 2010. https://www.dgzmk. de/patienten/faqs/zahnverfaerbungen-bei-kindern.html. Accessed 4 June 2018.
15. Elfrink ME, Ghanim A, Manton DJ, Weerheijm KL. Standardised studies on Molar Incisor Hypomineralisation (MIH) and Hypomineralised Second Primary Molars (HSPM): A need. Eur Arch Paediatr Dent 2015;16:247–255.
16. Temilola OD, Folayan MO, Oyedele T. The prevalence and pattern of deciduous molar hypomineralization and molar-incisor hypomineralization in children from a suburban population in Nigeria. BMC Oral Health 2015;15:73.
17. von Beck J, Eßer W, Gösling J, et al. Praktischer Ratgeber für die zahnärztliche Praxis. Frühkindliche Karies vermeiden. KZBV, BZÄK: Berlin, 2016. http://www.kzbv.de/ecc-ratgeber-einzelseiten-2016.download.78b1eb79e732ea8 b84fbd65a60ccbc60.pdf. Accessed 2 July 2016.
18. Viergutz G, Krämer N. Milchzahnverletzungen; zm online 2007;9. https://www.zm-online. de/archiv/2007/09/titel/milchzahnverletzungen/. Accessed 6 June 2018.
19. Drebenstedt S. Behandlung eines Dens invaginatus; ZWP online, 20.05.2011. https:// www.zwp-online.info/fachgebiete/endodontologie/fruehbehandlung/behandlungeines-dens-invaginatus. Accessed 23 July 2018.
20. Mossaz J, Suter V, Katsaros C, Bornstein, M. Überzählige Zähne im Ober- und Unterkiefer – eine interdisziplinäre Herausforderung. Teil 2: Diagnostik und therapeutische Konzepte. Swiss Dent J 2016;126:237–248.

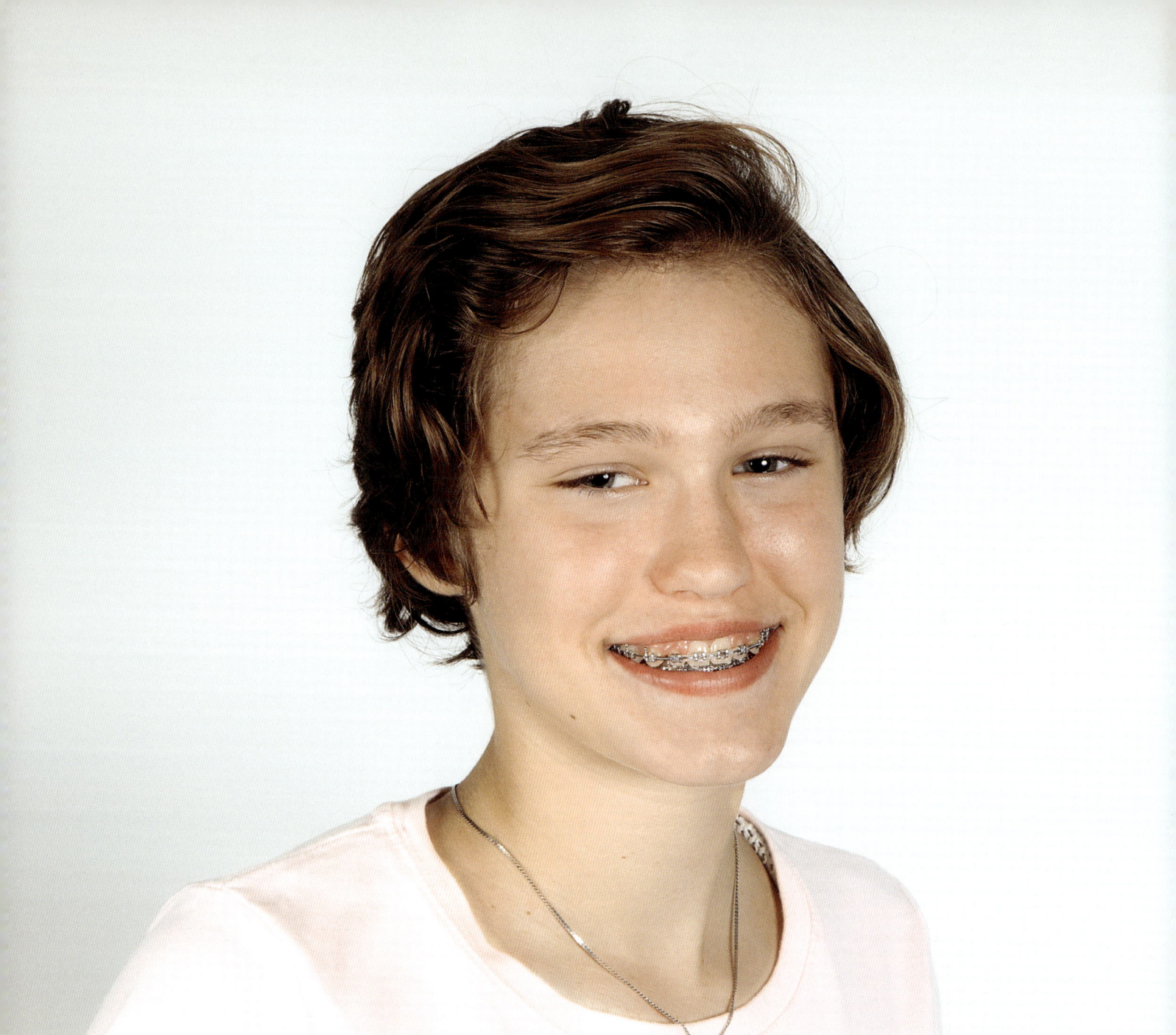

CHAPTER OUTLINE

7

TREATMENT CONSIDERATIONS AND APPROACHES

Because children are unable to take responsibility for their own oral and dental health, our job goes beyond just restoring defects. The far greater challenge of pediatric dentistry is to make parents aware of their responsibility, equip them with the necessary tools, and give them the motivation to safeguard our treatment results in the long term.

"We restore, you maintain."

ROBERTO MAGALLANES RAMOS

GENERAL ASPECTS OF TREATING CHILDREN

In principle, dentists should not apply a different standard to child patients and to adults. Working with the mindset that "they're just primary teeth" is not a maxim of quality-oriented dentistry. Persistent fistulae, leaving inflamed or open primary teeth as natural space maintainers, and using paraformaldehyde paste are obsolete methods without any scientific foundation.

Correct diagnosis is the most important thing in pediatric treatment. Unfortunately, lesions are often assessed too optimistically, or the diagnostic investigations are incomplete. Far too often, treatment begins on a child but results in failure because of inadequate diagnostics beforehand. The child is then referred to a specialist only when cooperation is unsatisfactory, which is a very unpleasant situation for everyone involved. Children need a definitive and age-appropriate solution. Before a decision is made to treat a child, the following points should therefore be considered:

- Caries rarely occurs on its own. Therefore, take radiographs (eg, bitewings) before starting conservative treatment.
- If the enamel marginal ridge (especially of the primary first molar) has broken down, endodontic treatment is likely to become necessary.

CAUTION ABOUT DEFECT ASSESSMENT

Do not be too optimistic when assessing defects. In the case of broken-down defects or active, whitish-yellowish carious lesions and interproximal defects, anesthesia is often necessary for a good treatment outcome.

- Methods such as selective caries removal in the primary dentition are possible in principle; however, absolutely tight restorations and hence very cooperative patients are required for these methods to be successful! On this subject, very good study results have been achieved, but mainly in a university setting and with appropriate case selection. Therefore, in the author's opinion, these results are not directly transferable to general dentistry practice.
- Are all necessary materials, such as stainless steel crowns, space maintainers, or Vitapex (NeoDental), available? Can the child be treated during the course of standard therapy, or is sedation necessary?
- When assessing treatment and selecting the therapy, it is important to bear in mind that children only tolerate a short duration of treatment. Five minutes' treatment time per year of life can be applied as a realistic rule of thumb.[1]
- Treatment should commence only when the dentist is certain that the child can be treated definitively in a child-appropriate manner and according to the indication. If not, it is more helpful to the young patient to be referred to a specialist immediately. This can be explained honestly and genuinely to the parents, who will understand and hence will not be dissatisfied.

A treatment plan should be drawn up before treatment is started. The following considerations should be incorporated in order to guarantee realistic treatment planning and avoid failure as far as possible:

TREATMENT-PLANNING CONSIDERATIONS
- **Depth of defect**
  - Superficial ⟶ No anesthesia
  - Deep (eg, broken-down enamel) ⟶ Anesthesia

- **Pain symptoms**
  - None ⟶ Normal filling placement
  - Stimulus-dependent pains, no nocturnal pain, no biting-down pain, pain only started recently ⟶ A pulpotomy might be possible
  - Nocturnal pain, spontaneous pain, biting-down pain, constant pain ⟶ Extraction; a pulpectomy might be possible if no interradicular radiolucency is present

⟶

- **Child's cooperation** (possibly referral to a specialist)
  - Very good ⟶ Standard treatment
  - Limited ⟶ Measures to increase compliance beforehand (carry out individual prophylaxis, desensitization measures), start with small defects, if possible; in case of doubt, **refer to a specialist before getting started**
  - None or severely limited and for minimal remedial effort ⟶ Arrest superficial lesions that are readily accessible to daily oral hygiene, for instance on smooth surfaces, by means of noninvasive measures (fluoridation, silver diamine fluoride [SDF]), regular checkups; measures to increase compliance through to definitive filling placement are possible; requires recall at short intervals and very good parental compliance; deeper lesions can be treated if the tooth and indication are appropriate
  - None or severely limited and for greater remedial effort ⟶ Different treatment techniques depending on the remedial effort required (see below), then refer to a specialist

- **Remedial effort** (possibly referral to a specialist)
  - Minimal (isolated fillings or possibly single-tooth extractions) ⟶ Standard treatment
  - Medium (several fillings, isolated extractions, and isolated endodontic measures) ⟶ Dependent on the patient's compliance and age: either standard treatment in which smaller, uncomplicated lesions are treated first and at the end extractions or endodontic measures are performed or, if compliance is slightly limited, using treatment aids in individual steps (nitrous oxide, sedation)
  - High (necessary invasive treatments in each quadrant) ⟶ With special treatment techniques such as sedation, nitrous oxide, or under endotracheal anesthesia

- **Tooth development stage** (based on radiographic imaging)
  - Shortly before tooth exfoliation ⟶ Extraction in the case of pain; otherwise no treatment
  - Root resorption more than one-third ⟶ No longer pulpotomy or pulpectomy because the potential for repair of the primary tooth pulp decreases with advancing resorption; ie, extraction in case of pain
  - Root resorption less than one-third ⟶ Pulpotomy or pulpectomy is possible

- **Child's age**
  - Infant ⟶ Take into account the attention span and the possible treatment duration as a consequence
  - The possible treatment time increases with age (depending on compliance)

⟶

- **Defect size**
  - Class I defect ⟶ Filling
  - Class II defect ⟶ Filling; for a very deep approximal lesion where the classic "box" preparation is not possible, preferably a crown
  - Larger than class II ⟶ Crown

- **Other considerations**
  - *Child's previous experience (possibly referral to a specialist):* Children with bad previous experiences will display limited compliance and in some circumstances it may be necessary to increase cooperation or employ different treatment techniques.
  - *Parental compliance:* Noninvasive treatment (fluoridation, SDF) of superficial carious lesions is only indicated if the parents are reliable in carrying out oral hygiene, can manage the child's diet and drinking habits, and attend regular recall visits at short intervals.
  - *Filling material:* Using cements in the masticatory area for class II defects might not be successful in the long term. Most children grind their teeth in the course of physiologic growing processes, which places fillings under greater stress.
  - *Dentist's experience (possibly referral to a specialist):* An important point that has a crucial influence on treatment outcome is the experience of the dentist. It is absolutely imperative for dentists to assess their skills realistically before starting treatment.

All these aspects should play a role in treatment planning and should therefore be taken into consideration. This is the only way to ensure a high success rate.

This chapter discusses all aspects of pediatric treatment. It is subdivided according to the invasive nature of the treatment, with the focus on conservative and endodontic treatment of primary teeth. Permanent teeth are only discussed specifically in the section "Dental trauma." The chapter concludes with the treatment of special cases encountered in practice, including primary molar hypomineralization, molar-incisor hypomineralization, trauma, the child as a pain patient, and antibiotic use in children (Fig 7-1).

Noninvasive treatment techniques
- Remineralization of initial dental hard tissue defects
- Fluorides
- Caesin phosphopeptide-amorphous calcium phosphate
- Silver diamine fluoride
- Other caries-preventive agents

Microinvasive treatments
- Caries infiltration
- Caries sealing
- Pit and fissure sealing

Minimally invasive and invasive treatments
- Nonrestorative caries control
- Terminal anesthesia in children
- Filling therapy
- Crown restoration in the primary dentition
- Basic principles of caries and endodontic treatment in children
- Surgical interventions

Particular challenges in everyday practice
- PMH and MIH
- Trauma to primary and permanent teeth
- Treating children in pain
- Antibotic use in children
- Sedation
- Treatment aids
- Cases that require referral to specialists

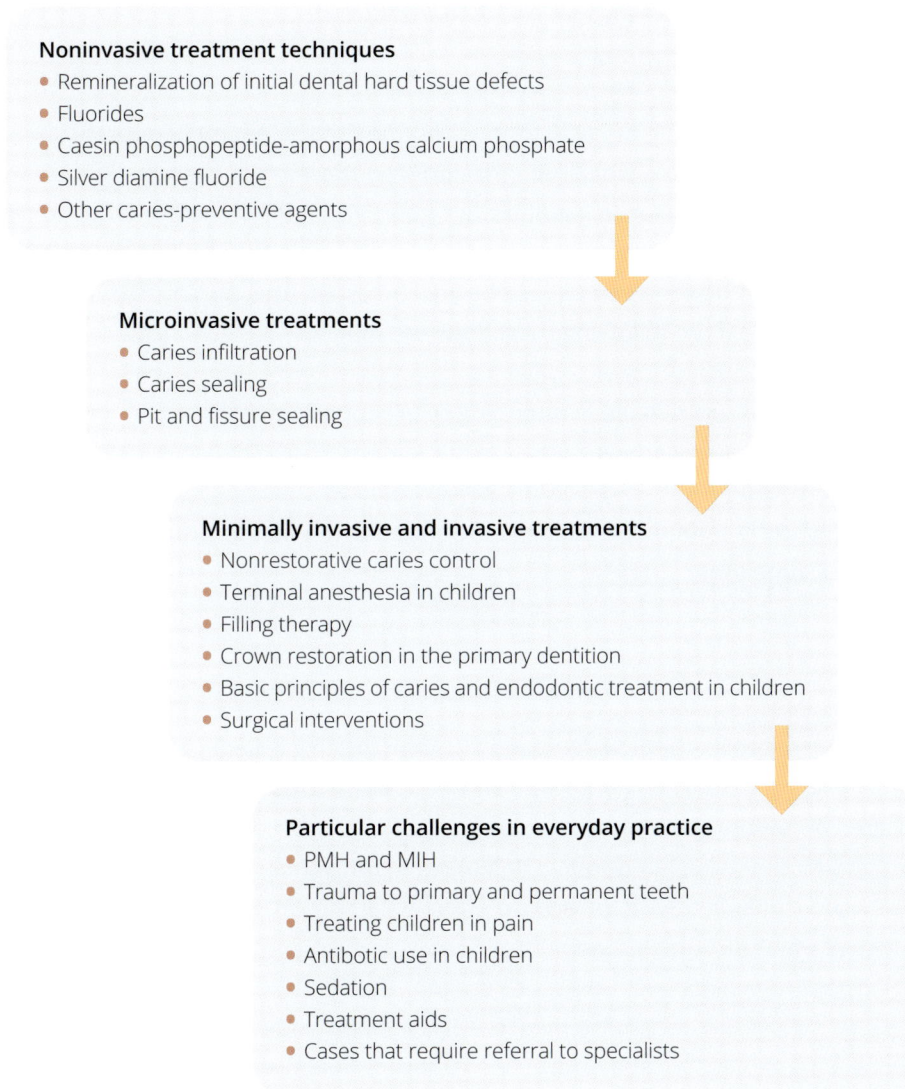

Fig 7-1 Overview of the structure of this chapter.

NONINVASIVE TREATMENT TECHNIQUES

Noninvasive treatment methods denote all prophylactic therapies as well as the noninvasive treatment of incipient caries.

Because children in the first and second year of life can have a very high risk of caries but are still too young to offer satisfactory compliance for standard dental treatment,[2] the focus must be on preventive measures: dietary and drinking advice to parents (see chapter 3), advice on oral hygiene (see chapter 3), the dental examination (see chapter 6), and, if applicable, treatment of the first carious lesions should be carried out.

REMINERALIZATION OF INITIAL DENTAL HARD TISSUE DEFECTS

Remineralization and arresting of initial lesions confined to the enamel are particularly important in pediatric dentistry. Not all initial lesions require invasive therapy right away, and more importantly, compliance is not always good enough for filling therapy to be performed immediately in young patients. Lesions confined to the enamel and readily accessible to daily oral hygiene can usually be well arrested. This noninvasive method should only be applied if the following conditions are met:

- The parents are entirely reliable in attending recall appointments
- Improvements in oral hygiene at home are implemented, and hence reliable plaque removal is achieved
- Other causal factors (mouth breathing, deficiencies in the diet or drinking) are eliminated at the same time.

PARENTAL INVOLVEMENT

Noninvasive caries therapy involves far more than treating lesions with fluoride or other preparations. This therapy can and will only be successful if parents are educated about the causes in detail. This makes thorough diagnostic assessment and history-taking imperative and leads to individualized, risk-oriented dietary and drinking advice, advice on effective and thorough oral hygiene, adjunctive myofunctional therapy if applicable, and, in some circumstances, other dental measures such as fissure sealing. Noninvasive caries treatment cannot be successful until these measures have been undertaken and all the other requirements listed above have been fulfilled. Noninvasive caries therapy is therefore closely linked to parental compliance, and the dentist must have an instinct whether this compliance exists. Frequent recall to check the treatment outcome is obviously essential in order to switch to invasive methods if there is any deterioration. The presence of initial lesions in infants suggests an increased risk of caries. Hence these children must be classified as high-risk patients and closely monitored accordingly.

The possible ways of assessing caries risk are discussed briefly below. The most common products used in the course of remineralization are then described.

Caries risk

Assessment of an individual's caries risk always involves identifying the prevailing risk factors. Because it is a multifactorial disease, various things need to be considered: low salivation rate, low socioeconomic status, unhealthy eating and drinking habits (highly frequent sugar intake), inadequate fluoridation, infection with *Streptococcus mutans*, the tooth surface (deep fissures, pits), caries experience, and plaque colonization, among other factors.[3]

In general dental practice, the question arises of which methods of caries risk assessment are suitable and effective and will also be accepted by the patient. Evidence of the risk of caries can, of course, be gained from microbiologic methods or saliva tests, but these methods are not really relevant to dental practices because of the costs involved. Testing for plaque is simpler, visually impressive, and more impactful in daily work with child patients and their parents (see chapter 3).

However, anyone wanting to use different methods for assessing the caries risk can utilize the "Dentoprog method" for primary school children. This method is suitable for children between the ages of 6 and 9 years. The individual caries risk can be estimated by the use of a slider and by recording the number of sound primary molars, the discolored 6-year molars, and the details of chalky-discolored smooth surfaces.[4] In the case of adolescents, a Cariogram, for instance, can be prepared.[3] The downloadable program is provided free of charge by Malmö University in several languages.[5] Certain parameters, tailored to the patient, can be entered into the program and used to produce a graphic depiction of that person's caries risk. In addition, the parameters can be altered to illustrate how the risk can be modified.

The clinical diagnosis of active and inactive carious lesions is, practically speaking, the most important aspect of caries risk assessment. Whether visually, radiographically, or by laser fluorescence, the caries risk can be established by determining the decayed, missing, and filled teeth (dmft) index (for primary teeth) or DMFT index (for permanent teeth). Based on this information, high-risk children can be identified (Table 7-1).[6]

TABLE 7-1 Definition of risk groups by age[6]

Age up to:	High caries risk if:
3 years	Not caries free, dmft > 0
4 years	dmft > 2
5 years	dmft > 4
6–7 years	dmft/DMFT > 5 or D(T) > 2
8–9 years	dmft/DMFT > 7 or D(T) > 2
10–12 years	DMF(S) on approximal/smooth surfaces > 0

*Children who meet the above criteria have a high caries risk. From the age of 10 years, the caries risk assessment is performed via smooth and approximal surfaces (DMF[S]).

EXAMPLE

If an 11-year-old patient, for instance, has buccal caries on the maxillary left first molar in a complete, otherwise caries-free dentition, the child's caries risk should still be assessed as high (since DMF[S] > 0; see Table 7-1).

FLUORIDES

Fluorides have been and continue to be the most important pillar of caries prevention. In recent years, pediatric dentists have increasingly found themselves confronted with parents and sometimes colleagues who are extremely confused about the effectiveness and hazardous nature of fluorides (see also chapter 3).

Fluoride is a trace element that occurs everywhere because it is found in bound form in nature and not in its elemental form because of its reactivity. Everyone ingests fluoride in different concentrations, depending on the individual diet. If fluoride intake is well-balanced, over 90% of this ingested fluoride is eliminated via the kidneys.

Fluorides inhibit demineralization and promote remineralization by inhibiting the carbohydrate metabolism of caries-causing bacteria, which thereby reduces acid production and the synthesis of extracellular polysaccharides. Fluorides react with the constituents of dental enamel and form fluoroapatite, which is more difficult to dissolve. They are also involved in the formation of a protective calcium-fluoride covering layer with calcium from the dental hard tissue or saliva.[7,8]

Fluorides have proved highly effective in the treatment of initial lesions and particularly in the prevention of caries. Fluorides can be used across a broad range of treatments at home and in the dental practice because they are available in a wide variety of forms, such as toothpaste, gels, and mouthwashes. Before giving a fluoride treatment, it is important to take a thorough fluoride history and to base fluoridation advice on the individual's caries risk.

Fluoride ions need to be continuously available in the oral cavity to achieve a caries-protective effect.[8] Where the caries risk is increased, oral hygiene at home with a fluoride toothpaste should be supplemented by intensive fluoridation as part of dental prophylaxis.

Four different fluoride compounds are used in caries prevention: amine fluorides, sodium fluorides, stannous fluorides, and sodium monofluorophosphate. These fluoride compounds all have their own areas of use. It is crucial to the effectiveness of fluoride application at home that the fluoride adheres to the tooth while using toothpaste. Amine fluorides adhere better to the tooth because the amine they contain acts as a surfactant, making the teeth more wettable. Furthermore, amine fluoride, even at lower dosages, forms a protective calcium fluoride layer more quickly than comparable fluoride compounds. Therefore, the use of amine fluoride compounds is advisable, especially in children's toothpastes that have a low fluoride concentration and short contact time on the tooth.

Recommendations for home fluoride application in high-risk patients

The following section deals solely with high-risk patients; for fluoride recommendations for children with a low risk for caries, see chapter 3. As the effect of caries prevention increases with the fluoride content of the toothpaste and cleaning frequency, patients with an increased risk of caries should undergo additional measures depending on their age.

Children

For children under 2 years of age, mouthwashes or long-term home use of high-dose gels are out of the question because this age group swallows nearly everything completely. Instead, twice-daily application of a smear of a fluoride-containing toothpaste (1,000 ppm in the morning and evening) promises a good caries-protective effect[2] (see chapter 3). In addition, the fluoride content of the drinking water should be checked, and any other sources of fluoride intake should be determined. In needed cases, consider prescribing a fluoride supplement. Children older than 2 years can switch to a pea-size amount of toothpaste.

For high-risk patients past their 4th birthday, the author recommends switching to a higher fluoride-concentration toothpaste to use in the evenings (1,500 ppm). Children should spit out excess toothpaste but must not rinse. Prescription-strength fluoride gels or varnishes are also available at most pharmacies, and these may be considered for children at especially high risk for caries provided the children can spit out well. Parents use a cotton-tipped applicator to apply a thin layer of the gel to the lesions concerned, and the fluoride is left to take effect. It can also be applied selectively with the aid of dental floss for interproximal defects. Any use of fluoride gel should be demonstrated to parents in the practice, and the success of the treatment should be checked at short intervals. By this means, cavitation can often be prevented and invasive treatments correspondingly delayed.

Prescription-strength fluoride gels or varnishes for home use in this age group should only be a temporary measure once a week for the duration of a month.[2] For high-risk patients older than 6 years, the American Dental Association (ADA) recommends a prescription-strength, home-use 0.5% fluoride gel or paste or 0.09% fluoride mouthrinse (www.ada.org/en/member-center/oral-health-topics/fluoride-topical-and-systemic-supplements).

Adolescents

For adolescents with a high level of caries activity, a prescription can be issued for toothpaste with a higher fluoride content (5,000 ppm) for daily use from the age of 16 years. Children with braces can also benefit from fluoride mouthwashes, which are available with different fluoride concentrations, in combination with fluoride toothpastes and the use of a fluoride gel once a week.[8]

Fluoride application in the dental practice for high-risk children

Studies have shown that younger patients at risk of caries can also benefit from several fluoride applications per year: Borutta et al wrote:

> "Higher-concentration fluoride varnishes can already be applied to nursery-age children because they dissolve very slowly. Provided they are applied expertly, the fluoride they contain only slowly gets into the body. Therefore, higher-concentration fluoride varnishes are toxicologically harmless if used properly. It was even shown in a recent study that punctate application of a
>
> ⟶

higher-concentration fluoride varnish to the anterior teeth in infants with an increased caries risk can delay the development of caries."[8]

High-risk patients, irrespective of age, should therefore be called in for follow-up and individual prophylaxis every 3 months. Application of highly concentrated fluoride preparations four times a year in the form of varnishes or gels is safe and useful in infants and nursery-school children.[2] Four applications of fluoride varnish before the age of 2 years will reduce decay by up to 30%. The ADA recommends 2.26% fluoride varnish for children younger than 6 years and 2.26% fluoride varnish or 1.23% fluoride (acidulated phosphate fluoride) gel for patients 6 years or older (www.ada.org/en/member-center/oral-health-topics/fluoride-topical-and-systemic-supplements). Care should be taken to ensure that the preparations are able to dry briefly on the teeth after application before the child closes his or her mouth. In addition, this approach can guarantee early loyalty to the dental practice.

EVIDENCE ON FLUORIDE
Of all the popular caries prevention products, fluorides have by far the highest evidence level.

CAESIN PHOSPHOPEPTIDE-AMORPHOUS CALCIUM PHOSPHATE

Casein phosphopeptide-amorphous calcium phosphate (CPP-ACP) is mainly found in chewing gums or as a paste.[9] Recaldent is a common commercial name (Mondelez). The available studies are inconclusive, but products containing CPP-ACP appear to promote remineralization of the enamel. As the remineralization process is also linked to the presence of calcium (calcium fluoride surface layer), these products can help to arrest and remineralize incipient caries defects.

The use of these products has proved effective in dental practices, mainly to treat hypersensitivity in structurally damaged teeth (ie, primary molar hypomineralization [PMH] and molar-incisor hypomineralization [MIH]). Pastes are available in a variety of flavors, and they are well accepted by children and parents alike.

After brushing their teeth in the evening, affected children can apply a pea-sized quantity of CPP-ACP paste to the damaged teeth and leave it to take effect for at least 5 minutes. For severe forms of MIH, home use of Recaldent products worn in a splint for 20 minutes is another possibility. One advantage, especially in view of the increasing number of convinced opponents of fluoride, is that the remineralizing effect is achieved without fluoride. Admittedly the evidence for this is rather weak. Nonetheless, CPP-ACP products have proved effective in practice, and studies suggest that this effect is stronger if fluoride is applied at the same time.

CAUTION ON CPP-ACP

CPP-ACP products must not be used on children with a milk protein allergy. Their evidence is much less than that of fluoride, but in practice their use has proved particularly helpful in the treatment of hypersensitivity linked to PMH or MIH.

SILVER DIAMINE FLUORIDE

The use of silver diamine fluoride (SDF) is also an effective method for arresting initial carious lesions, which has recently come more strongly into focus. Until now, SDF has mainly been used in developing countries or for economic reasons. It offers a few advantages: It is quick to apply, it requires minimal cooperation, it can be applied to smooth surfaces and even into interproximal spaces with the aid of Super Floss (Oral-B), it is cost-effective, it is a delegable procedure, and it is reliable in exerting its effect of arresting multiple, quickly progressing carious lesions. A major drawback is the black discoloration of treated lesions so that an esthetic treatment outcome cannot be achieved. It is imperative to tell parents about this before the treatment. For this reason, SDF is often described as "third world dentistry"—quite wrongly in the author's opinion.

Undoubtedly this therapeutic approach is not right for every patient. The fact remains, however, that SDF can very reliably arrest caries with minimal effort and low treatment costs. As a result, it gives the dentist time to increase the child's cooperation, for instance, to safely bridge the waiting times for endotracheal anesthesia or sedation appointments, or even reduce a high level of caries activity. SDF has an antibacterial action, thereby inhibiting bacterial growth.[10] The 38% solution is recommended for single and localized use (hence confined to the affected tooth/teeth). Twice-yearly treatment (every 6 months) has demonstrated an unmistakably preventive effect.[11] Many dentists use it at 3-month intervals, while others apply it before placing a provisional or definitive restoration.

When SDF is being used, care should be taken to cover clothing and surfaces carefully because it can stain surfaces and leave marks on skin or mucosa. These usually disappear from mucous membranes within 2 weeks. The product must not be applied to large areas in the mouth because it can irritate the mucosa. Furthermore, any allergy to the ingredients definitely must be ruled out beforehand. The use of SDF is additionally contraindicated in the case of ulcerative gingivitis, aphthous stomatitis, during pregnancy, and for breastfeeding mothers. There has been increasing research with this substance recently, and it remains to be seen whether SDF preparations become a serious alternative to tried and tested topical prophylactic measures. However, preliminary results are extremely promising. Clinically it has been used extensively for years with very good results.

Application of SDF is described in the package leaflets of the particular products, but it is generally straightforward:

1. Protect the mucous membranes with gauze or cotton wool rolls positioned lingually and buccally.
2. If appropriate, apply petroleum jelly to protect the mucous membranes.
3. Dry the tooth concerned.
4. In the case of occlusal or broken-down interproximal caries, open the cavity wide enough to be able to apply the SDF and, if possible, avoid undercuts (even possible with hand instruments); if possible, gently remove soft carious parts with a hand instrument prior to SDF application.
5. For interproximal caries that has not broken down the tooth surface, guide the fluffy part of Super Floss under the interproximal contact and brush the product onto this part of the floss—this will absorb the fluid so that the product actually gets to the interproximal defect.
6. Apply the product very sparingly (1 drop only), let it take effect for 60 seconds, and then disperse the excess with air or rinse off or remove with a cotton wool roll.

It is imperative to remember that even the smallest areas of demineralization, for instance on adjacent teeth, will discolor on contact with SDF. In such cases it may be advisable to use petroleum jelly to isolate visible surfaces of neighboring teeth, for instance, in the anterior dentition.

SDF can also be used for sealing fissures on incompletely erupted molars of children with a high level of caries activity. It is also suitable for use in patients who are physically or mentally disabled or very young with early childhood caries (ECC), for example. It can additionally be utilized to treat hypersensitivity of MIH teeth. Use of SDF would also be justified for arresting root caries in geriatric dentistry.

Black-discolored surfaces can—but do not necessarily have to be—covered with a filling (glass-ionomer cement [GIC] or even adhesive materials). The black discoloration will often show through the eventual filling. However, there is no reason why discolored areas cannot be removed and an esthetic filling placed at a later date when compliance is better. Advantage Arrest (Elevate Oral Care) is a great product to use.

CAUTION ON SDF
SDF should only be used on symptom-free teeth without pulp exposure.

SMART technique

In the United States, where SDF has been in use for years, the objective is often a combination of SDF and minimally invasive filling therapy, together known as the *SMART technique* (silver modified atraumatic restorative treatment). The base ART technique

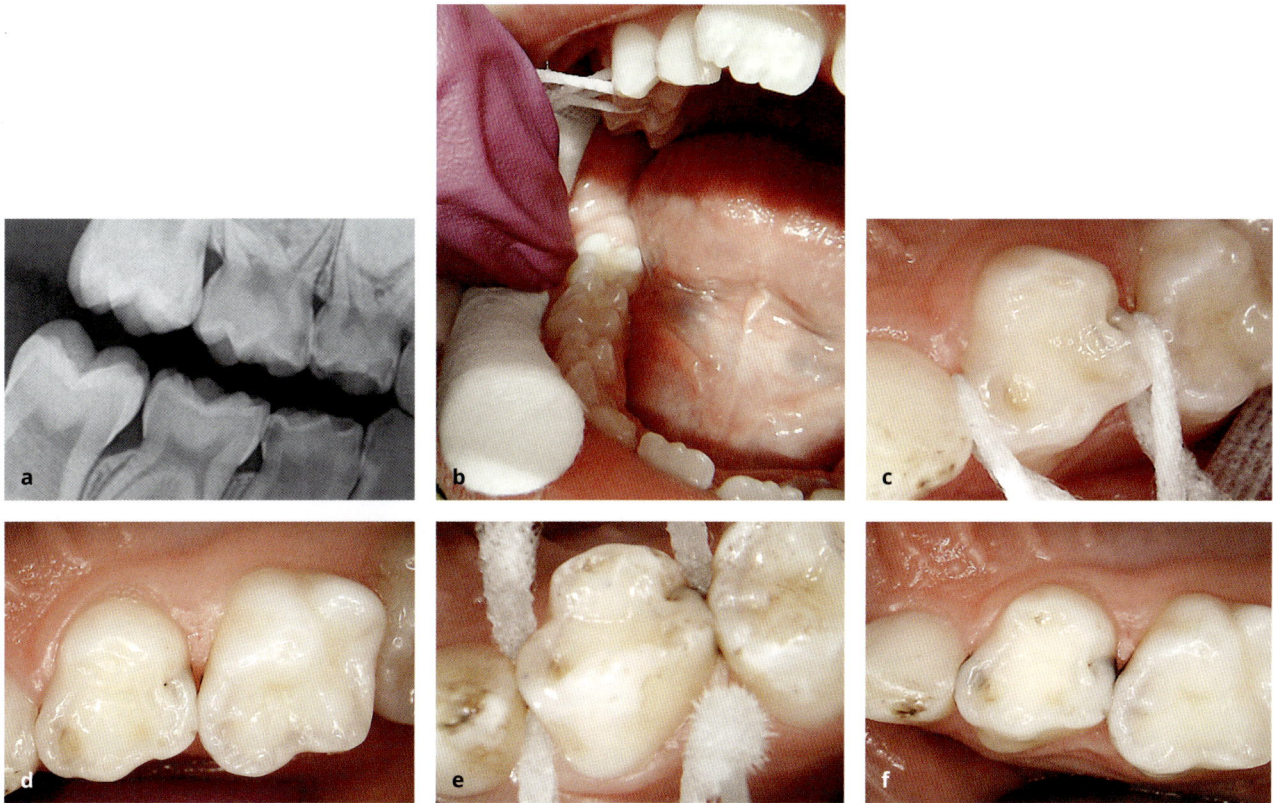

Fig 7-2 *(a)* Bitewing radiograph of the right quadrants at the start of treatment. The patient is an early teether and 5 years old at the time of treatment. *(b)* Introduction of Super Floss dental floss and isolation with saliva pad and cotton wool rolls in the maxilla. *(c)* Position of the Super Floss. *(d)* Result of staining after SDF application. *(e)* The second SDF application (2 weeks after the first application). The preparation is applied very sparingly (1 drop) to the soft portion of the Super Floss dental floss with a tuft, so that the SDF is absorbed. *(f)* End result after a total of three SDF applications.

involves incomplete caries removal (usually just with hand instruments) followed by filling treatment, usually with GICs.[12] It is pain-free for little patients and hence is well accepted. The SMART technique involves applying SDF after hand excavation but before filling placement.[13,14] The SDF application and subsequent restorative treatment can be done in a single session or in two separate sessions for patients with limited compliance.

Like other approaches, these SDF techniques are undoubtedly not suitable for every patient. Nevertheless, they do expand our range of treatments and provide other options for acutely treating selected patients, without the use of endotracheal anesthesia or similar, so that standard treatment can be accomplished by means of desensitization and behavioral change.

Figure 7-2 demonstrates interproximal SDF application in several noncollapsed lesions, and Fig 7-3 demonstrates application by the SMART technique to a deeper interproximal lesion. At the time the treatment was started, the 5-year-old patient was not cooperative enough for all the lesions to be restored with fillings. With the aid of SDF treatment, caries was arrested while gradual desensitization was carried out, eventually permitting at least temporary filling placement with GIC at the mandibular right primary first molar.

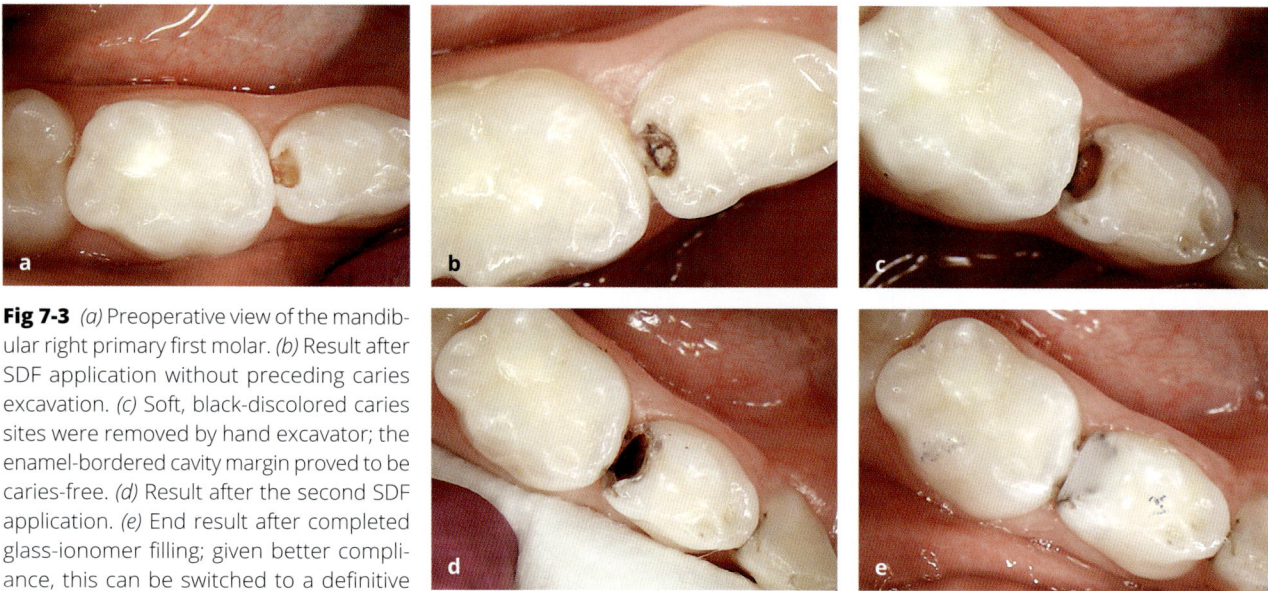

Fig 7-3 *(a)* Preoperative view of the mandibular right primary first molar. *(b)* Result after SDF application without preceding caries excavation. *(c)* Soft, black-discolored caries sites were removed by hand excavator; the enamel-bordered cavity margin proved to be caries-free. *(d)* Result after the second SDF application. *(e)* End result after completed glass-ionomer filling; given better compliance, this can be switched to a definitive compomer or composite filling.

OTHER CARIES-PREVENTIVE AGENTS

As well as the above-named active agents, other preparations are used for caries prevention. However, the level of evidence for these preparations is low, and they should therefore be used only as a supportive measure and never on their own for caries prophylaxis, especially in high-risk children.

Chlorhexidine digluconate

Chlorhexidine digluconate (CHX) can demonstrably reduce the quantity of plaque. Nevertheless, CHX can only be used once children are definitely able to spit it out and will readily accept the bitter taste. CHX is suitable, for instance, for short-term use if sufficient oral hygiene is not guaranteed.

Xylitol

Xylitol has a caries-inhibiting effect because it intervenes in the bacterial metabolism of *Streptococcus mutans*. Xylitol is added as a sweetener to various products, such as chewing gum, sweets, and other confectioneries, but it is also available as a gel or powder. The level of evidence for caries inhibition by xylitol is highest for chewing gums, but these seem unsuitable for children under 3 years because most of them cannot yet chew gum safely. Furthermore, a high frequency of application is required (up to six times a day; total dose up to 10 g) to achieve a therapeutic effect. For high-risk children under 3 years, Thumeyer and Schlüter recommend taking a xylitol lozenge four times over the course of the day (a total of 5 g xylitol) in conjunction with application of xylitol gel to the teeth before bedtime, in addition to daily oral hygiene with a children's fluoride toothpaste.[2]

It should be noted that xylitol can have a laxative effect if more than about 0.5 g per kilogram body weight is ingested. This should be explained to parents.

CAUTION ABOUT XYLITOL

The use of products containing xylitol should be carefully considered in terms of nutritional physiology and primarily in terms of health education. Frequent consumption of sweet products has a lasting effect on how our children's sense of taste develops.[15] Parents must not forget to make it clear to their children that a xylitol lollipop is actually a sweet. If (small) children have unrestricted access to tooth-friendly sweets, they will learn just one message: "sweets are okay." Primary school children cannot distinguish between a lollipop containing xylitol or a normal lollipop, so encouraging xylitol-containing candies as healthy or good is not a good approach in the author's opinion. Furthermore, there has been a rapid increase in food intolerance in recent years. There is evidence from nutritional scientists that the increased quantities of sugar consumed by children and the frequent use of sugar substitutes encourage the development of fructose malabsorption disorders and their associated complaints. This subject also requires detailed explanation to parents and responsible handling of the product.

Arginine

Arginine is an amino acid that has been shown in studies to speed up neutralization of the pH and thereby exert a caries-protective effect. Basic Bites (Ortek) is a promising arginine product that is even suitable for younger children and can also be recommended as an excellent substitute for classic sweets. The recommended daily intake is two Basic Bites.

Probiotics

Probiotics are microorganisms that can shift the oral balance in favor of a protective flora where harmful microorganisms compete for the environment. The basis is that colonization, particularly in the first 3 years of life, can reduce the growth of caries-causing bacteria. The best-known and best-researched strains are lactobacilli and bifidobacteria. Probiotics can be found in foods such as yogurts but also as drops or tablets. In America, for instance, there are probiotics specially formulated for dental use in the form of lozenges. A few studies on preschool children suggest that, with the use of probiotics, it might be possible to reduce caries in primary teeth[16] by increasing the saliva buffer capacity and by driving out bacteria that cause caries.[17] However, the reviews on this subject agree that the level of evidence is still low and more comparable clinical trials are needed for really reliable recommendations to be made for dental practice.[18,19] As yet this approach should only be viewed as a complementary measure.

MICROINVASIVE TREATMENTS

Microinvasive treatments include caries infiltration, caries sealing, and fissure sealing.

CARIES INFILTRATION

Caries infiltration can be used to treat interproximal defects that have not broken down as well as initial carious defects on smooth surfaces, for instance after bracket removal. The basic principle of the treatment is that the infiltrant, a highly fluid resin, is "drawn" into the carious lesion by capillary action, fills it up, stabilizes it, and cuts off diffusion pathways for cariogenic bacteria.[20] On smooth surfaces, there is an added esthetic benefit; as the resin infiltrant has a similar light refraction index to intact enamel, extremely esthetic masking of initial defects can be achieved.

This treatment technique requires very good compliance from the child because a rubber dam is essential and the waiting time between the separate steps is not inconsiderable. Furthermore, the patient must attend recall regularly and reliably in order to guarantee the success of the treatment. A helpful tool is the Icon radiograph holder system (DMG America), which makes it possible to repeat bitewing radiographs in a reproducible position to verify the treatment outcome.[21] Because Icon is not radiopaque, it is all the more important to obtain comparable radiographs. This is why patients should also be given an Icon patient logbook to guarantee complete documentation in case there is a change of dentist.

Undoubted advantages of caries infiltration are that it is gentle on dental hard tissue and causes no pain during the treatment. The esthetic aspect when treating initially carious smooth surfaces is also highly appealing.

> **NOTE ON CARIES INFILTRATION**
> Carious lesions in the enamel region can be treated by means of caries infiltration. It is no longer indicated once carious lesions encroach on the first third of the dentin.

After cleaning, once the teeth are absolutely dry (and when treating interproximal defects after separation), apply the Icon etching gel for 2 minutes. Rinse this off with water for 30 seconds and dry the tooth. Then apply an alcohol, Icon Dry, and let it take effect for 30 seconds before drying with air again. Next apply Icon infiltrant and wait 3 minutes for it to take effect. This is followed by light curing for 40 seconds and final polishing and removal of excess.[20]

Because of the time required to complete this procedure and the high costs involved, the risks and benefits should be very carefully weighed when considering caries infiltration, particularly in infants with high caries activity. Nonetheless, a few studies on caries infiltration applied to primary teeth show that this method is a promising treatment alternative for preventing the progression of interproximal caries.[22–24] Admittedly the amount of data available is still very small.

ICON FOR ENAMEL DEFECTS OF DIFFERENT ORIGIN

Icon can also be used to mask enamel defects on teeth. For a good result, some practitioners recommend performing mechanical enamel microabrasion before the Icon protocol. This entails applying a hydrochloric product that contains some abrasive particles as well (eg, Opalustre, Ultradent; it contains 6.6% hydrochloric acid combined with silicon carbide particles). After the mechanical abrasion, the Icon procedure can be started and carried out in the recommended way. It can be necessary to repeat the etching part (which is a chemical abrasion) or the infiltration step depending on the appearance of the lesion.

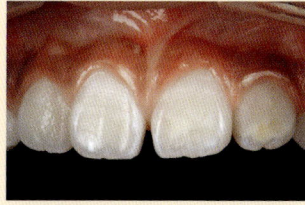

1. Anterior teeth before the treatment.

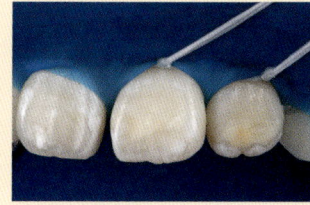

2. Applying rubber dam.

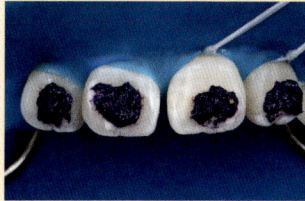

3. Microabrasion using Opalustre and a polishing brush or rubber cup. This is an optional step.

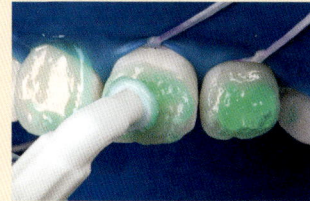

4. Applying Icon Etch. It is possible to repeat this step.

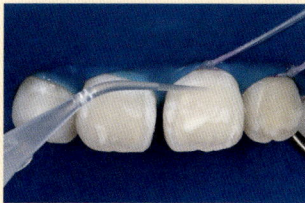

5. Applying Icon Dry.

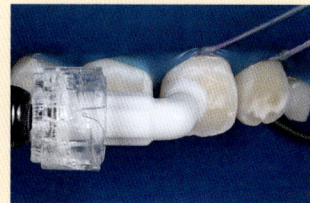

6. Applying the Icon Infiltrant.

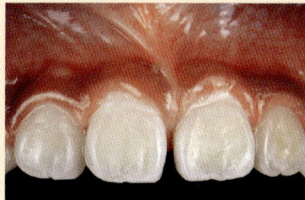

7. The enamel changes could be successfully masked, thus improving the esthetics.

All photographs courtesy of Dr Jorge Casián Adem.

In the author's opinion, caries infiltration is not really a serious treatment option for primary teeth. It demands a high level of compliance from the child and, on that basis, there are other effective strategies for treating interproximal caries in primary teeth. For permanent teeth it is indeed an effective, gentle, and, above all, esthetic measure.

CARIES SEALING

Caries sealing refers to covering superficial, noncavitated caries on an occlusal surface by means of sealing. Sealing with a filling material—similar to infiltration—creates a diffusion barrier with the aim of cutting off the existing cariogenic bacteria from any supply of substrate.[2]

The basic requirement for success is an absolutely tight restoration, which should be checked regularly. This does not necessarily have to be an adhesive restoration. Especially in very small children, superficial occlusal defects can also be sealed with GICs in order to prevent caries progression. The dentist gains time to eliminate caries-causing factors, for instance, and to establish a certain degree of compliance. However, crucial factors in the success of this method are the diagnostic assessment (no cavitated dentin lesions!), the tightness of the restoration, and the reliability of the parents in attending recall appointments regularly. That means this method must be weighed very carefully and is definitely not suitable for every patient.

FISSURE SEALING

Classic pit and fissure sealing is a widely used caries-preventive measure. The evidence level for its use in the primary dentition to prevent ECC is low, and it seems only advisable in exceptional situations.[25] In the permanent dentition, sealing should not be done to all molars in a sweeping fashion. For children with a very low caries risk, sealing of permanent molars is only recommended if they are morphologically so difficult to clean that a locally increased risk of caries will result. Fissure sealing is indicated, however, as a preventive measure for children with active caries.[26]

If the dentin is already affected, the caries first needs to be excavated. Incompletely erupted molars should not be sealed or at least not with composites because it is not possible to achieve an adequate dry field. In the case of high-risk children or structurally damaged teeth, erupting molars, or patients with low compliance, modified GICs (eg, Fuji Triage, GC America) may also be used. Figure 7-4 provides a helpful decision-making algorithm.[26]

An adequate dry field must be guaranteed for the clinical procedure of fissure sealing with low-viscosity composite. The prerequisites are basic cooperation from the child, working in a four-handed system, and, if some work is delegated to the chairside assistant with prophylaxis duties, the use of rubber dam. However, because rubber dam placement is difficult or impossible, especially if there is no undercut, and is often not accepted by children, at least four-handed working is required. This can help to ensure an adequate dry field. After cleaning fissures with fluoride-free prophylaxis paste and a rotary brush, condition the surface with 35% phosphoric acid (1 minute on a permanent tooth and 2 minutes on a primary tooth) in order to obtain a retentive etching pattern.

For extended fissure sealing that involves the dentin, 30 seconds' enamel etching followed by 15 seconds' dentin etching are required. Then apply the low-viscosity resin sealant bubble-free and set according to the manufacturer's instructions. To guarantee

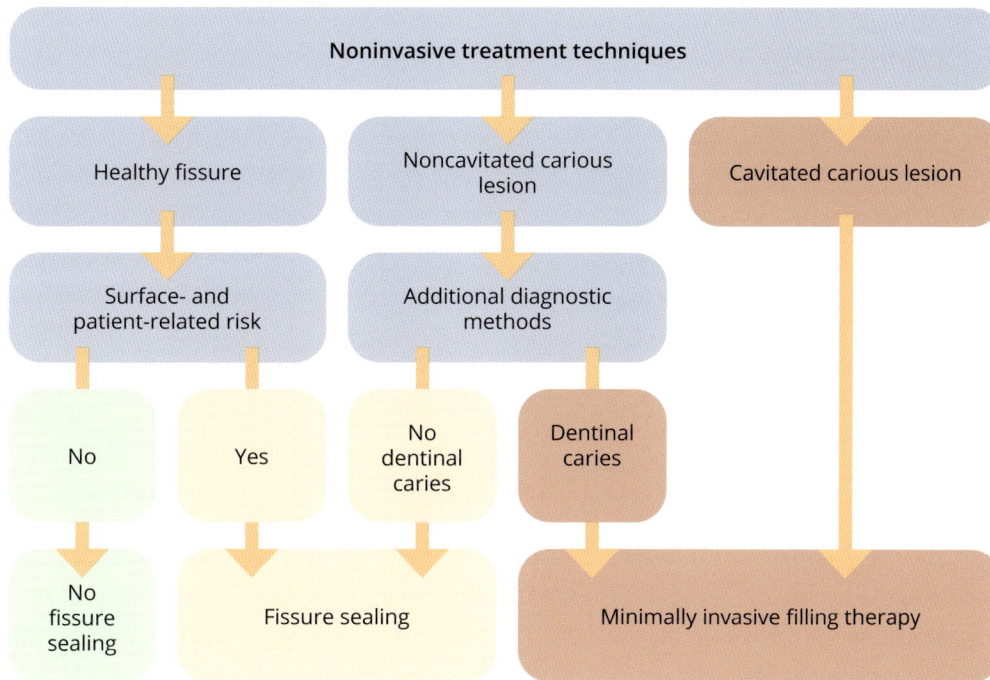

Fig 7-4 Algorithm for the treatment of carious lesions.[26]

complete setting, especially with opaque resins, it is imperative to adhere to the specified time, depending on the lamps used. The material should be applied thinly and without excess. After occlusion has been checked, polishing must be performed to remove the incompletely set oxygen-inhibition layer on the surface. Finally, a fluoride varnish should be applied for remineralization.

MINIMALLY INVASIVE AND INVASIVE TREATMENTS

All measures involved in caries and filling therapy are discussed here. This includes an explanation of the different filling materials, crown restoration in the primary dentition, and possibilities of caries and endodontic treatment. A basic precondition for the success of these measures is that pain is sufficiently eliminated, which is why a detailed discussion of the subject of anesthesia appears in this section.

Furthermore, extractions and surgical interventions are discussed. The following tips on treating children are intentionally as practical as possible in order to guarantee the utmost success even for nonspecialist colleagues. Special forms of treatment (nitrous oxide, sedation, endotracheal anesthesia) should be left to colleagues specializing in pediatric and adolescent dentistry.

TREATING CHILDREN
Treating children can be demanding and challenging, especially for those with little experience. This is why it is all the more important to assess one's own skills realistically before starting in order to avoid lengthy or repeatedly unsuccessful treatments, which would lead to reduced patient compliance and would cause parents to lose confidence in the dentist. If you decide to treat children in your practice, your treatment principles should be based on the most up-to-date knowledge.

NONRESTORATIVE CARIES CONTROL

Nonrestorative caries control refers to superficial exposure of carious lesions (creating access to the lesion and removing undercuts) with the aid of rotary or hand instruments (eg, exposing interproximal defects from the occlusal direction). As a result, the carious sites become accessible to daily cleaning, and the caries can be arrested with selective application of fluoride. Nonrestorative caries control resembles the SMART approach (see earlier section titled "SMART technique") except that fluoride agents are used instead of SDF. Suitable restorations can be placed as a second step but are not necessarily carried out.[27] The teeth must not exhibit any pulpal involvement and should hence be pain-free. The method can be used when patient compliance is limited in order to slow down and/ or halt caries progression and to limit the loss of dental hard tissue. Once again, it is true that this method will certainly not suit every patient, but it can work extremely well with selected children and parents and result in a high level of patient satisfaction. In a study from 2015, this method demonstrated a slightly better chance of success than conventional filling therapy, but it performed rather worse than the Hall technique.[27] It should be noted that this method can only be successful if the parents carry out thorough oral hygiene at home and attend regularly for recall appointments. The parents need to receive detailed instructions on oral hygiene. Particularly with uncooperative children, it may thus be possible to bridge waiting times until anesthesia appointments or maybe even avoid the need for endotracheal anesthesia. It might also enable the dentist to gain enough time to improve compliance so that restorations can be prepared.

TERMINAL ANESTHESIA IN CHILDREN

Before classic filling therapy in the primary dentition is addressed, an important basic prerequisite for successful invasive treatment in children needs to be examined: dental anesthesia. Successful treatment of children often depends crucially on whether pain is satisfactorily blocked. It is extremely important to make use of local anesthesia, especially in children. Primary teeth have large pulps, and children can feel pain during caries removal even with small defects. The consequences of neglecting pain elimination are the typical failures of pediatric treatment: poor cooperation from children, resulting in large areas of residual caries being left in place, consequently increased loss of fillings, and multiple treatments of a single tooth—all in all, an unsatisfactory treatment outcome for all concerned, which will do nothing to promote patient loyalty. As a result of experiencing pain, little patients often refuse to cooperate at all, and yet many dentists are reluctant to give them an injection. There is no reason for this; on the contrary, it greatly simplifies treatment and increases the success rate. The following tips are intended to help dentists overcome their inhibitions.

With topical anesthesia, a little distraction with a made-up story, slow (!!!) injection and use of the finest injection needles (eg, from an intraligamentary anesthesia system), and a tightly stretched vestibulum for buccal infiltration are usually straightforward enough to provide a child with adequate pain elimination. Absolutely crucial to a successful terminal anesthesia is time. The topical anesthesia must be allowed about 3 minutes to set, and the injection itself should be done very slowly. After injection, we must wait for 5 minutes before we get started. Another possibility to make it more comfortable for the patient is to warm up the capsules to body temperature. Of course, computer-aided anesthesia (eg, The Wand, Milestone Scientific) is an option for anesthetizing without pain. However, this form of pain elimination is nowhere near standard in dental practices, purely because of the very high purchase costs. With satisfactory terminal anesthesia, any treatment—no matter what—will be far more relaxed for everyone and can be performed without interruption.

Occasionally, terminal anesthesia is not enough when treating primary mandibular molars in children over the age of about 6 years. In this case, the teeth need to be numbed with a nerve block or by intraligamentary anesthesia. Especially for children and bearing in mind bite injuries, the use of intraligamentary anesthesia is recommended and is preferable to classic nerve block. Studies show that intraligamentary anesthesia is also an alternative to nerve block for endodontic treatments.[28]

In the author's view, nerve block is almost never indicated. Before anesthesia, the altered sensation should be explained to young patients. Sentences such as "Then you won't feel anything" should be avoided because it is not really true and it can cause children to stop the treatment repeatedly as they can still feel something. This is rarely a matter of feeling actual pain but instead a confusion between pain and vibration. It is better to make it clear that the sensation will just be altered: pain will be removed but the patient will still be aware of vibration and pressure.

Intraligamentary anesthesia systems are well suited for pediatric dentistry because they do not have the typical appearance of a syringe, which children associate with vaccinations, for instance. With Citoject (Kulzer), for example, children can be distracted if they are told to join in counting the clicks while the injection is being given. Even if a practice does not have an intraligamentary anesthesia system, very fine and short cannulas can also be used for classic infiltrative anesthesia. This makes the puncture less painful. In any event, local surface anesthesia of well-dried oral mucosa can be helpful beforehand. It should be injected slowly without pressure while the vestibulum is kept tightly stretched. If an extraction, pulpotomy, or pulpectomy is planned in the maxilla, palatal anesthesia must also be given. Intraligamentary anesthesia following vestibular infiltration is often more pleasant than palatal infiltration anesthesia in the maxilla. If an intraligamentary system is not available, Viergutz and Hetzer recommend transpapillary anesthesia prior to the palatal puncture: "To do this, the injection needle is guided slowly through the interdental papilla from buccally as the anesthetic is steadily released. Only then is another injection of approximately 0.2 mL anesthetic given from the palatal side into the pre-anesthetized mucosa."[29] This method works extremely well and can also be used with intraligamentary anesthesia because, here too, the first palatal puncture to the tooth is thoroughly unpleasant for a lot of children.

Intraligamentary anesthesia should be applied to plaque-free teeth and is contraindicated for patients at risk of endocarditis.

TIPS FOR ADMINISTERING ANESTHESIA TO CHILDREN

- Remember to communicate with the child and explain what is happening in a child-friendly way (see chapter 2). Before administering any anesthetic, explain that you're about to put the teeth to sleep, so you need to get everything ready, like the pajamas, the cozy bed, etc. Explain that you're going to dry the cheek before putting some sleeping drops on the teeth to make them go to sleep. Show the child the Citoject without injection needle. After handing the device back to the dental assistant so that the needle can be attached, dry the mucosa and apply the surface anesthesia gel, commenting on how good it smells (eg, "Don't you think it smells like raspberry ice cream?"). Tell the child to close his or her eyes to show the teeth that it's time to go to sleep. This gives the dental assistant the opportunity to hand over the anesthetic under the headrest without the child seeing the needle. While slowly (!!!) injecting, talk to the child in a soft, monotone voice, saying something like: "You're doing great; your little tooth is slowly getting tired and putting his pajamas on." Go into detail about the tooth's pajamas or make up other elements of the story that can distract and amuse the child as the injection is being given, for example, how the tooth is snuggling under the covers or shutting its eyes. Count the clicks together as you administer the anesthetic, always encouraging the child that he or she is doing well. After counting the clicks together as the "sleeping drops" are administered, tell the child that when you count to 10, the teeth will be asleep and the child can open his or her eyes again. Start counting to 10, and be sure to have handed the anesthesia system back to the assistant before you reach 10 so that when you do, you can immediately tell the child that the teeth are asleep: "You did really, really well. Can you tell there's now a little pillow in your cheek? It feels magical, doesn't it?" You can then have the child rinse with water, and if any blood is visible, explain that the last few drops were red-colored, so the spit might be a little red.

→

- In the author's practice, the child is told that there's a contest to see who counts the most drops, and the winner gets an extra prize. After administration of the anesthesia, the child is asked how many drops they counted, and then the dental assistant pretends to look up the rank. Sure enough, the child is then told that "Wow, you won the first prize. Congratulations! That means you can pick an extra prize today at the end of the treatment." This method works extremely well to keep the child focused on counting and distracted from what's going on.
- With very anxious or restless children, it may be advisable during the anesthesia for the dental assistant to hold an arm in the air above the child's upper body. This can prevent the patient's arms from suddenly lifting up. In addition, it is important to maintain physical contact. The dental assistant's hand may rest gently on the shoulder or the tummy of the patient. The assistant should NOT stroke the child. Anesthetic that is running off should be removed by suction because children often find its bitter taste very unpleasant and, in some cases, it can cause the treatment to be interrupted.

Anesthetic doses for children and choice of anesthetic

Generally speaking, the available substances are very well tolerated. Taking a thorough general medical history will, of course, minimize the incidence of complications, as in adult patients. It is also clear that the maximum dose must be respected. Articaine is suitable as a local anesthetic. It has very good bone penetration and provides better pain elimination than lidocaine.[30] Incidentally, articaine is also recommended as the anesthetic of choice for pregnant and breastfeeding women (due to high plasma protein binding and the short half-life).

According to Daubländer and Kämmerer,[30] "the metabolization of articaine is not influenced by the patient's age," which means that calculation of the limit dose is not age-independent. It is 7 mg/kg body weight for solutions containing adrenaline and 4 mg/kg bodyweight for adrenaline-free solution. The maximum dose is calculated as follows:

$$\text{Maximum quantity (mL)} = \frac{\text{maximum dose (mg/kg)} \times \text{weight of patient (in kg)}}{\text{concentration of solution (mg/mL)} \times 10}$$

The concentration details are given in the product information. The usual concentrations for dental local anesthetics are 4% for articaine, 3% for mepivacaine, and 2% for lidocaine.[31]

Calculation example: The articaine preparations of Ultracain (Sanofi Aventis) are always in 4% solution. This means that if the child weighs 10 kg and an adrenaline-containing anesthetic (maximum dose = 7 mg/kg body weight) in a 4% solution is used, the calculation is as follows: 7 mg/kg × 10 kg divided by 4% × 10 (ie, 70/40). This gives 1.75 mL maximum quantity, which equates to one anesthetic cartridge. In the case of an adrenaline-free solution (maximum dose = 4 mg/kg body weight), the maximum dose is 1 mL (calculation: [4 × 10] / [4 × 10] = 1), which is slightly more than half an anesthetic cartridge.

Most children with 10-kg body weight are aged 1.5 to 2 years. This means that if the dentist is treating an older patient, the child's body weight is probably much higher. One cartridge of adrenaline-containing 4% articaine solution (eg, Ultracain DS or Ultracain DS Forte) can generally be used in properly developed children with an unremarkable history.

Nevertheless, the dentist should take care to follow the manufacturer's instructions. Ubistesin (articaine product from 3M), for example, should only be given to children from 4 years of age according to the manufacturer.[32] In the case of Ultracain, the only note in the product information is that the anesthetic has not been tested in children under 12 months.[33]

CAUTION ABOUT ANESTHESIA

Surface anesthesia must be taken into account when calculating the maximum dose. This should merely be applied in a punctate manner to the dry mucosa, rather than over an extensive area. The recommended exposure time is about 1 minute.[29]

FILLING THERAPY

Fundamentally, several factors are crucial to successful filling therapy in the primary dentition: tooth type (hence the first or second dentition), child's age, compliance, how long the tooth will remain in the oral cavity, caries activity, and tooth position.[34] Several factors should also be taken into account when choosing the material. If the level of caries activity is high and cooperation is poor, GIC is definitely a good temporary choice. Compomers or composites should be used in the case of good compliance, and stainless steel crowns should be used for very extensive defects.[34]

GENERAL TIPS ON FILLING THERAPY
- If defects are too extensive, filling therapy is unsuitable, and they should be restored with a crown.[35,36]
- For primary teeth that will remain in the mouth for several years, all types of cement are unsuitable as a definitive filling material in class II cavities and have by far the highest loss rates.[37-40] For class I cavities, GIC fillings achieve better retention rates.[41]
- Preparing definitive restorations without a matrix is not an appropriate treatment. T-band matrices, for instance, are well suited to conservative treatment in the primary dentition (Fig 7-5). They can be adapted to any size

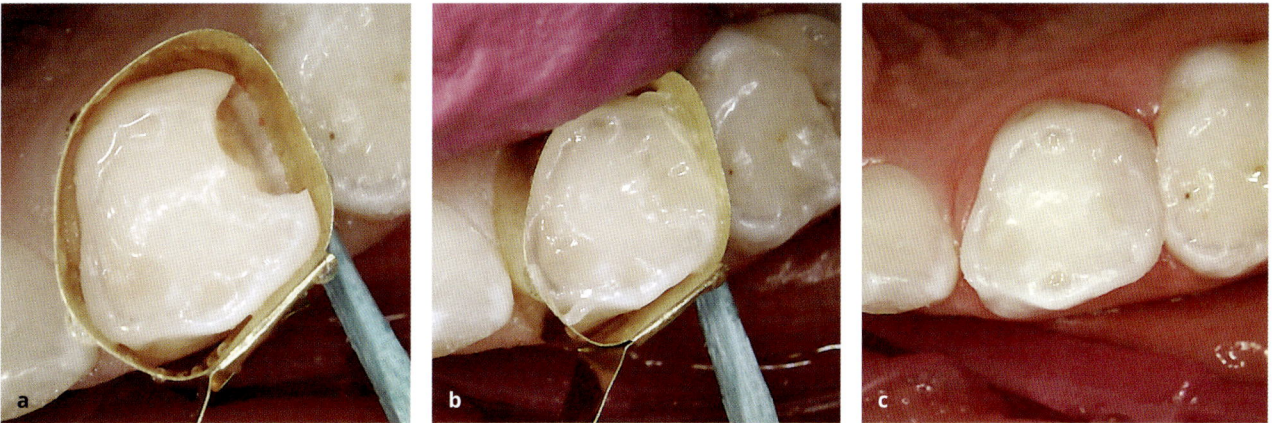

Fig 7-5 *(a)* T-band matrix in place and wooden wedge for restoring a primary molar. *(b)* Compomer filling (Dyract, Dentsply) immediately after light curing. *(c)* Finished filling.

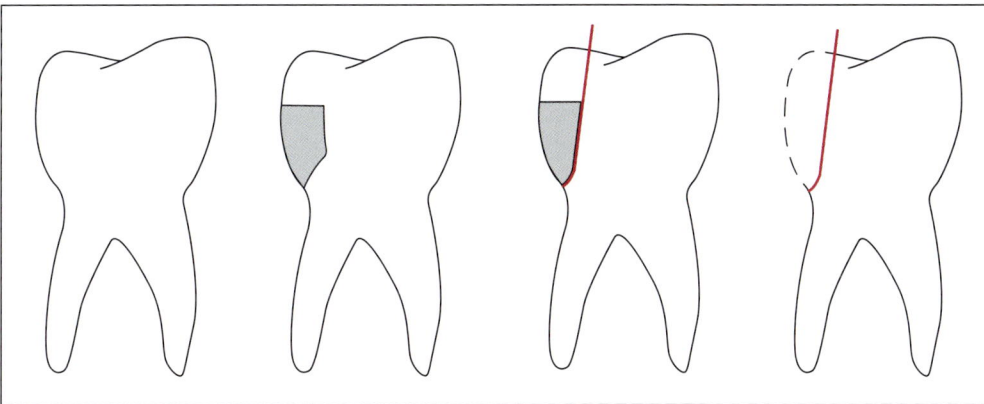

Fig 7-6 A shoulder cannot be prepared because of the approximal extent of the caries.

of primary tooth, they are thin, they can be easily contoured, and they can be made palatable to the child as a "gold medal for the tooth." Other systems, especially with partial matrices, are extremely well suited to the restoration of primary teeth. In an article from 2004, Krämer and Frankenberger also recommend Tofflemire ring band matrices with a small contoured band.[42] BiTine rings (Dentsply) are also a great tool to achieve tight contact points.

The interproximal areas are often so heavily affected by caries that, after caries removal, there is no longer a remaining interproximal shoulder because of the pronounced taper of the primary teeth (Fig 7-6). In these cases, increased filling losses and/or fractures can occur, making it necessary to restore the lesion with a crown.

Material selection for primary teeth

How long a filling lasts in the primary dentition is not solely dependent on the material. Practitioner-associated factors have a major influence—ie, selection of the right filling material that takes into account not only the patient but also the defect and processing of the particular material. Overall care of the patient and the child's successful engagement with routine prophylactic recall are crucial factors. Filling therapy will not achieve sustained success if caries activity is not sustainably reduced, regardless of which material is used.

The American Association of Pediatric Dentistry writes in its guideline on restorative therapy in the primary dentition:

> "It is now recognized that restorative treatment of dental caries alone does not stop the disease process, and restorations have a finite lifespan. Conversely, some carious lesions may not progress and, therefore, may not need restoration. Consequently, contemporary management of dental caries includes identification of an individual's risk, understanding the individual patient's development of caries, and active observation in order to estimate the progression of the carious lesions and, with appropriate prophylactic measures plus filling therapy, if indicated, to control the development of caries."[43]

The decision on which filling material to use should be made according to the following:

- Size of the defect
- Compliance of the child and parents
- Caries activity and the patient's caries risk
- Further treatment planning (if endotracheal anesthesia is planned)
- Timing of the restorative work in relation to exfoliation
- The context in which the treatment is taking place (eg, while GIC is contraindicated for restoration of primary teeth in the context of endotracheal anesthesia, standard treatment may nevertheless be advisable with limited compliance)

As in adult patients, the aim should be to provide our little patients with appropriate, long-term dental rehabilitation. In fact, standard restoration (ie, the fabrication of definitive restorations in the masticatory area of cooperative children) of primary teeth with GIC or composite-reinforced GIC is not a lasting and qualitatively appropriate restorative approach for young patients. Krämer and Frankenberger wrote 16 years ago: "It is still striking, however, that materials which function in the permanent dentition as long-term temporary restorations, at best, are being supplied particularly for primary teeth restoration."[42]

As yet very little has changed, and temporary filling materials are seen as standard by some practitioners when treating primary teeth. There are certainly indications for GIC in primary tooth filling therapy, but it should never be the rule for definitive filling of typical class II defects in cooperative patients. There are now various studies that document the durability of various filling materials in children and provide a good starting point for selecting the right material. Higher rates of filling losses or fractures due to secondary caries or due to the wrong filling material can and should be avoided. To achieve this, careful treatment planning is required (see "General Aspects of Treating Children" at the beginning of this chapter).

Composites

When using composites it is important to know that primary teeth are structured differently to permanent teeth (see chapter 1). The aprismatic enamel layer of primary teeth covers a dentin layer, which is less well mineralized and has enlarged dentinal tubules. Nevertheless, good retention rates are possible, although the success of composite restorations depends on compliance with the very sensitive application protocol.

Krämer and Frankenberger wrote that the "vulnerability of composites to cooperation-related errors is very striking."[42] With regard to conditioning of the primary tooth enamel, the authors write:

> "It is advisable to bevel the primary tooth enamel as widely as possible because of the aprismatic surface. Etching with 30% to 40% phosphoric acid for 30 seconds after removal of the aprismatic enamel surface is adequate. Owing to the micromorphologic characteristics, however, dentin should not be etched for longer than 10 seconds. The risk of over-etching is that the primer might not be able to cover the increased distance to the unchanged, non-demineralized dentin. The result is hydrolytic degradation of the non-hybridized collagen fibers after a certain amount of time. Minimally invasive preparation can generally be carried out when restoring class II cavities with composite. However, the adhesive technique is only possible in the case of interproximal involvement if no compromise in treatment needs to be made. Cavity lining should be ignored in favor of total bonding."[42]

A dry working field and strict adherence to the manufacturer's instructions, especially regarding the use of adhesives, are crucial to the success of composite fillings. A clinical trial from 2016 further suggests that composite restorations exhibit better and more durable marginal adaptation if etch-and-rinse bonding systems are used or if the primary tooth enamel is still classically etched beforehand in self-etch systems.[44] No advantage of multiple-bottle systems has been demonstrated. The problem with all clinical trials is the very short follow-up period, making it difficult to obtain really workable statements. In addition, there are only a few comparable study designs.[45]

No advantage of composites over compomers has been reported in the literature. Composites achieve the same success rates in the primary dentition, but their application is far more sensitive, and they require excellent compliance from the child.

COMPOSITES OVERVIEW

Composites can function in the primary dentition with class I and II cavities, provided they are applied correctly with a very good dry field (rubber dam). As adhesive systems, multiple-bottle systems offer no advantages, although bonding is better with etch-and-rinse systems than with self-etch systems. When the latter are used, additional prior etching with phosphoric acid should be performed to improve marginal adaptation, or the primary tooth enamel should at least be beveled widely in order to remove the aprismatic portion.[42] Composites are ruled out as a filling material for very agitated children or those with limited cooperation.

Compomers

Especially in Europe, compomers seem to be the method of choice for conservative restoration of primary teeth.[46] This is because they are simpler to handle than composites, yet they offer tooth-colored esthetics, the possibility of minimally invasive preparation, and long-term superiority over GICs or resin-reinforced GICs in terms of fracture susceptibility, for instance. An added factor is that compomers release fluorides and hence have a caries-protective action. This fluoride release is constant over a lengthy period of time and is not initially increased as it is with GICs.[47] Compomers therefore combine the good properties of composites with those of GICs. Cavity lining can again be omitted in favor of adhesive bonding.

To improve the bond, these materials should be used with an adhesive system. It should be noted that use of the acid-etch technique when filling with compomers in the primary dentition does not provide better retention than the use of a single-bottle dentin adhesive. The latter is hence adequate when using compomers.[48] Compomers were originally intended for use without an adhesive. Studies clearly showed, however, that use of compomers without bonding agents dramatically reduces the success of fillings.[37,38] By implication, this means that a child with average cooperation can be treated with a compomer, provided the dry field is guaranteed for the bonding and filling process. An absolute dry field with the use of rubber dam is not necessary.

COMPOMERS OVERVIEW

For children with average cooperation, compomers are particularly suitable for ensuring long-term success in the restoration of class I and II cavities. Phosphoric acid etching of the enamel does not have to be carried out. However, the use of a single-bottle adhesive should not be omitted. A relatively dry field is adequate, and cavity lining is not necessary. Compomers are preferable to GICs and composite-reinforced GICs for definitive filling placement in sufficiently cooperative children. Compared with composites, there are no drawbacks; in fact, the use of compomers is easier and quicker.

$\longrightarrow$

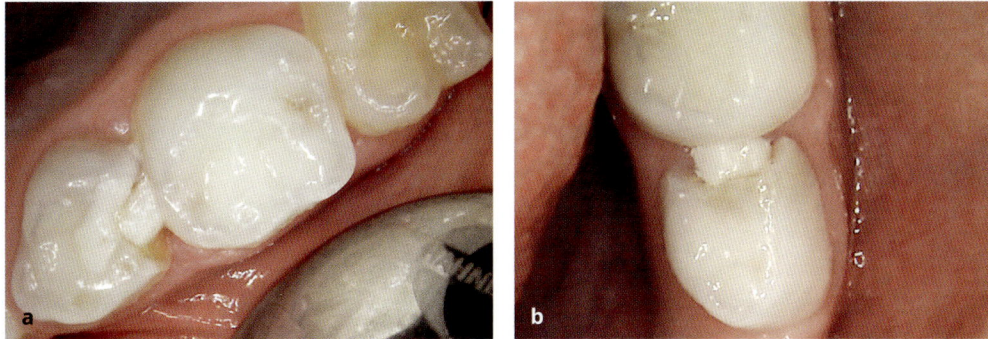

Fig 7-7 *(a and b)* Two broken and inadequate GIC fillings in primary molars in an 8-year-old boy. The fillings were prepared 3 months before by a different dental practitioner.

Tip: The purchase of a compomer may still be worthwhile, even if only a few children attend the dental practice for filling therapy. This filling material is ideally suited to treating root caries in older patients.

GIC and resin-modified GIC

GIC or resin-modified GIC is often used for definitive primary tooth fillings. However, practical experience shows that these materials are not really suitable for long-term, definitive filling therapy. Especially when restoring class II cavities, the fracture risk is enormous, and the success rates are poor (Fig 7-7). A lot of dentists actually use GICs because of the fluoride release and the associated caries-inhibiting effect. Unfortunately, this effect does not come into play because of the short survival time of glass-ionomer fillings.[42]

The clinical results are only slightly improved with resin-modified GICs, but they are still markedly inferior to compomers. Furthermore, a few of these materials release high levels of monomer.[49]

GICs as well as resin-modified GICs cannot compete esthetically with compomers; they are also much rougher on their surface. Despite these drawbacks, (resin-reinforced) GICs have a perfectly justified range of indications and have become an integral part of pediatric dentistry. Especially in very young patients whose cooperation is poor due to their age, GICs can serve temporarily as a filling material. It is important to explain to parents that this is a temporary solution that can be switched to a definitive restoration with a different material at a suitable date when the child is more compliant.

Furthermore, GICs are also ideally suited to sealing erupting 6-year molars in very caries-active children. Definitive fissure sealing can be performed once the teeth have fully erupted and an adequate dry field is created. In the case of patients who are very uncooperative or have physical or mental disablilities, the molars can be protected in this way, at least until eruption is fully completed.

In addition, the use of GIC has proved effective as temporary protection of MIH molars. Affected molars are often highly sensitive to cold and touch. The consequence is that thorough oral hygiene of these teeth, in particular, remains undone. Because it is extremely difficult to create a dry field here, especially during the period of eruption, temporary restoration with GIC can at least minimize the risk of fracture of the teeth and reduce hypersensitivity in these children. This in turn contributes a great deal to the increased compliance of these children.

> **GIC OVERVIEW**
>
> GICs are extremely well suited as temporary filling materials. The 6-year molars can be temporarily protected with GIC in patients with very active caries or MIH. In the author's opinion, GICs or resin-modified GICs are rather unsuitable for long-term filling treatment of primary teeth with class I or especially class II cavities in cooperative children.

Amalgam in children?

Restoration with amalgam is a matter of growing controversy. While amalgam is still used routinely in other countries,[43] the EU Commission decided that from July 2018 amalgam must no longer be used in pregnant women and children in Europe.[50] The issue certainly needs to be discussed critically and in an unbiased way. Are composites really less or not at all harmful? There is in fact evidence that certain BPA derivatives can pose a health risk.[43] Two major clinical trials did not reveal any risk to the health of children who had been treated with amalgam.[51,52] An added factor is that amalgam fillings exhibit much better durability than composite fillings.[53] The survival rate of amalgam fillings is twice as high as that of GIC or resin-reinforced GIC. Only compomers can compete with amalgam fillings in durability.[37,38] In view of these facts, we should still guard against replacing existing, intact amalgam fillings in children.

CROWN RESTORATION IN THE PRIMARY DENTITION

The indication for a crown must be established more quickly in pediatric dentistry than with adult patients. This is partly due to the specific shape of the primary teeth (cervical marginal bulge, which is often involved in approximal caries) and partly due to the broad pulp, which often requires an endodontic measure during the course of caries therapy and finally makes a crown restoration necessary.

Basically, prefabricated crowns are the only option for primary molars, stainless steel crowns being differentiated from tooth-colored zirconia crowns. In addition, restorations made from composite and strip (Frasaco) crowns can be prepared for the anterior teeth. Table 7-2 summarizes the pros and cons of stainless steel and zirconia crowns for primary teeth.[54]

TABLE 7-2 Advantages and disadvantages of different primary tooth crowns

Type of primary tooth crown	Advantages	Disadvantages
Steel crown	Easy to place, good retention	Esthetics
Veneered steel crown	Esthetics improved	Dimensionally stable, no individualization possible, great loss of tooth substance, wear of the acrylic resin veneer
Zirconia crown	Esthetics	Dimensionally stable, no individualization possible, great loss of tooth substance, no long-term experience

Data from Lauenstein and Sieper.[54]

Prefabricated stainless steel crowns

Prefabricated stainless steel crowns (SSCs) are an excellent alternative for simple restoration of primary teeth that is not unduly user-sensitive. Many colleagues in general dentistry shy away from this treatment yet have no problems spending hours fabricating complex prosthetic work for their adult patients. Why is that? This type of restoration is easy to learn and is ideal for treating extensive defects, restoration of endodontically treated teeth (see below), and cases of poor compliance (see section "Hall technique") and high caries activity. Hypomineralization disorders can also be treated very well by this method.

> **TIP FOR USING SSCs**
> When "daring" to attempt an SSC for the first time, it is important to select an uncomplicated young patient for the purpose. The primary maxillary first molars occasionally have a very pronounced vestibular marginal bulge at the neck, which can make it far more difficult to adapt the crown. Furthermore, the vestibulopalatal dimensions of the maxillary first molars are usually large, whereas the mesiodistal dimensions are rather narrow. In such cases it can be difficult to select the right crown. Primary second molars or primary mandibular first molars are definitely more suitable for gaining initial experience of using prefabricated SSCs.

If they are correctly used, SSCs can offer several advantages when integrated into one's practice concept:

- Children can receive definitive remedial care in just a few steps.
- No risk of filling loss.
- No risk of secondary caries.
- High level of patient and dentist satisfaction.

The indications for restoration of primary teeth with prefabricated SSCs are the following:

- Primary molar hypomineralization and associated defects
- Restoration after endodontic treatments (pulpotomy and pulpectomy)
- Extensive fillings (three-layered)
- High caries activity
- Limited cooperation
- Deep interproximal defect so that there is no longer a cervical shoulder

The Hall technique, ie, restoration of a primary tooth with an SSC without prior preparation, is first discussed below, followed by classic SSC preparation.

Hall technique

This technique originates from Scotland and is named after the dental surgeon Dr Norna Hall. While this option for treating caries, which is minimally invasive and preserves pulp vitality, is not yet widely used in the United States, studies suggest that this restorative alternative is not only readily accepted by patients and parents, but it is also very popular with dentists (particularly colleagues in general dentistry).[55] Furthermore, the Hall technique has higher success rates than conventional filling therapy.[56] Therefore, it is definitely worth seriously engaging with this treatment option, even for specialist colleagues.

In the Hall technique, prefabricated primary tooth crowns made of stainless steel are fixed with GIC without anesthesia, without prior caries removal, and without any preparation of the tooth. As a result of the absolutely tight seal, the caries bacteria perish because of the lack of substrate, thereby arresting the development of further caries. The technique naturally has to be explained to parents beforehand. The crowns should also be shown to parents and children. Like other treatment options, it is clearly important to establish the correct indication, strictly observing the following criteria:

- The teeth concerned must not have any pulpal involvement, which means an intact dentin bridge to the pulp must be present according to radiographs, and the tooth must not be sensitive to pain or percussion.
- The Hall technique is strictly contraindicated if there is any pulpal involvement, in caries profunda, in the case of noticeable radiographic features (resorption, interradicular radiolucencies) or pain, etc. If there is any uncertainty on this point, temporary restoration with GIC is first recommended, followed by 3 months' waiting time, then restoration by the Hall technique if the tooth is symptom-free.[34]
- Absolutely uncooperative children or patients with immunosuppression or endocarditis must not be treated by this technique.

The Hall technique offers a broad range of indications and is user-friendly because neither preparation nor anesthesia is required. Thus, good restorative work can be done in one or two sessions, even with anxious children. It can be used for the following:

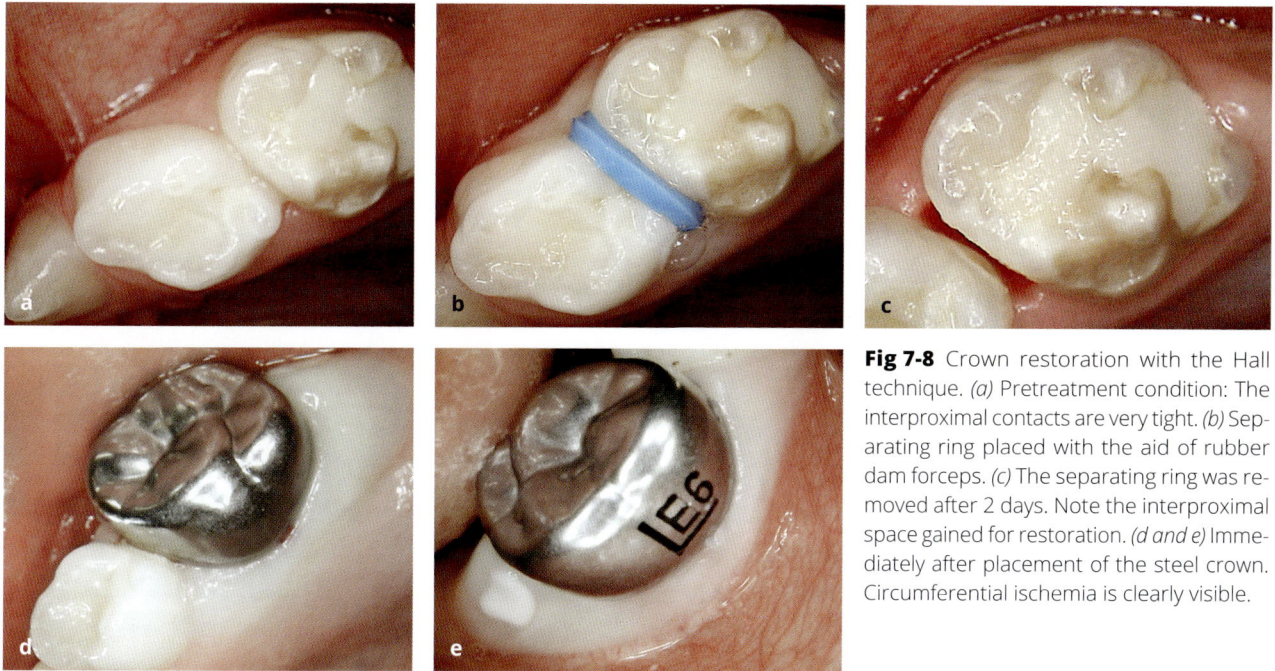

Fig 7-8 Crown restoration with the Hall technique. *(a)* Pretreatment condition: The interproximal contacts are very tight. *(b)* Separating ring placed with the aid of rubber dam forceps. *(c)* The separating ring was removed after 2 days. Note the interproximal space gained for restoration. *(d and e)* Immediately after placement of the steel crown. Circumferential ischemia is clearly visible.

- Carious primary molars with two or more involved surfaces
- Primary molars that are badly damaged by hypomineralization disorders or that are very sensitive to pain
- Children with increased caries activity
- Very anxious children who are moderately cooperative but will not tolerate conventional treatment with anesthesia, filling placement, etc

After thorough diagnostics, including radiographs, first select the smallest possible crown; all the cusps should be covered, and the crown should meet resistance approximally when slightly pressed down. If interproximal contacts are very narrow (30% to 50% of patients), it may be necessary to insert separating rings 2 to 3 days beforehand with the aid of rubber dam forceps or with dental floss so that the crown can be placed in a second session.[57] The teeth can, of course, be separated interproximally using a diamond, depending on the cooperation of the child being treated. Fill the crown up to the margin (!) with low-viscosity GIC, then press onto the tooth concerned.[58] Dentists can either get a child to bite closed or press on the crown themselves with a finger. Remove excess cement, including interproximally. In the best case, the crown comes to lie in a subgingival or at least an equigingival position. The accompanying ischemia of the gingival margin usually subsides after a few minutes.

Figure 7-8 shows the restoration of a hypomineralized primary second molar by the Hall technique and prior separation with a rubber ring. The tooth was still hypersensitive and at risk of fracture despite a previous GIC filling.

Fig 7-9 *(a)* Temporary increase in vertical occlusal height after placement of a steel crown by the Hall technique. *(b)* Regular occlusion observed 1 week after cementation of a Hall crown.

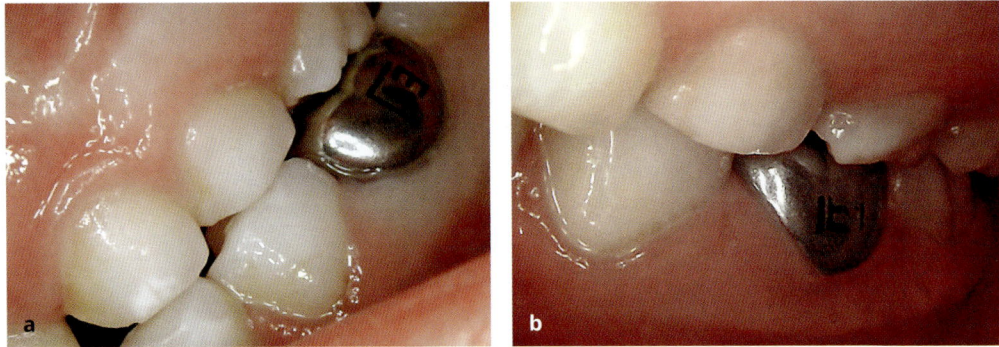

TIP FOR THE HALL TECHNIQUE

Analyze the exact morphology of the tooth in advance. The primary second molars are better suited for first use of the Hall technique because they often have favorable mesiodistal and orovestibular dimensions. An excellent guide to the Hall technique with illustrations, case studies, literature references, and suggestions on problem management is available free of charge from the website of the University of Dundee.[58]

When the Hall technique is used, the bite is temporarily raised by about 2 mm (Fig 7-9a). This usually causes children an altered sensation in the first 24 to 48 hours. It is therefore important to explain to patients beforehand that it might take 1 or 2 days for the tooth to get used to the new "princess crown" or to the new "knight's armor." There are no negative consequences of this temporary bite raising documented in the short or long term in the literature. The vertical increase in the bite is no longer detectable after a few days[57] (Fig 7-9b).

In a study from 2007, acceptance of the technique among dentists, parents, and children and the success rate were tested versus conventional composite restorations. The results speak for themselves and have been confirmed in more recent studies from 2014. In their study, Innes et al[55] restored a total of 128 teeth using the Hall technique and examined the restorations after 23 months; 89% of the teeth exhibited only very mild or no unpleasant sensations (versus 78% of teeth with composite restorations), and only 1.5% caused unacceptable discomfort (4.5% for composite fillings). Also, 77% of the children, 83% of the parents, and 81% of the dentists preferred the Hall technique to composite fillings as a better restorative technique. At follow-up of the restorations after 23 months, the teeth restored by the Hall technique performed better than teeth with composite fillings: Irreversible pulpitis was found in 2% of the Hall teeth and 15% of the composite restorations; progressive caries or loss of retention affected 5% of the Hall teeth and 46% (!!!) of those restored with composite; and pain occurred with 2% of the Hall teeth and 11% of the control restorations with composite.[55] Equally good results were achieved by Santamaria et al in a clinical trial from 2014 with a follow-up period of 1 year.[57]

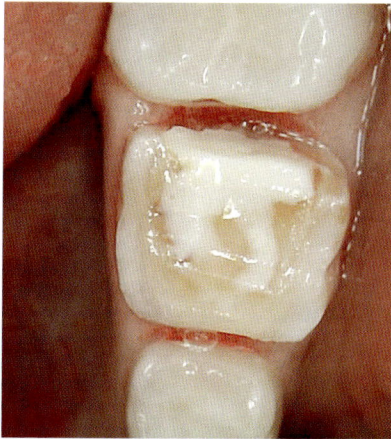

Fig 7-10 Occlusal reduction by 1.5 mm and interproximal separation without shoulder formation with rounded edges on the mandibular primary second molar to receive an SSC. Due to a hypomineralization disorder of the primary molars, there was repeated occlusal fracturing of the tooth and severe sensitivity to cold, so restoration with an SSC was indicated. Previous fillings were fractured time and time again.

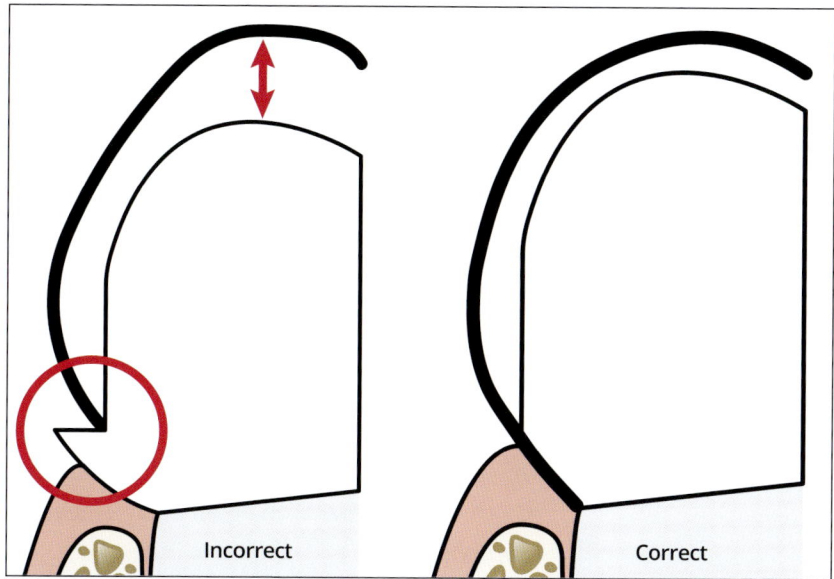

Fig 7-11 Principles of interproximal preparation to receive an SSC. Shoulderless interproximal preparation is important for an absolutely tight crown margin, ideally lying subgingivally. (Courtesy of Drs Sabine Dobersch-Paulus and Stefanie Feierabend.)

The Hall technique can therefore be recommended as a simple and promising method for restoring primary teeth. Even for specialist colleagues, this technique is entirely recommendable for selected children and may be considered a viable option.

Classic SSC preparation

The great advantage of SSCs is the fact that they adapt to the natural anatomy of primary teeth and hence require minimal preparation. The elastic feather edge of the preformed crowns snaps over the cervical enamel bulge, ensuring a tight seal with shoulder-free preparation. Preparation is remarkably simple and can be done in three steps:

- First perform occlusal reduction by about 1.5 mm, provided it is still necessary after caries excavation. Some publications advocate recreating the occlusal relief with a bur during reduction, but in practice this is not necessary. Flat height reduction is entirely adequate (Fig 7-10). Instead of making sure to reproduce the tooth anatomically correctly in the preparation form, it is more important to work speedily, carefully, and purposefully to avoid unnecessarily overtaxing the young patient's compliance.
- This stage is followed by approximal separation by means of tangential preparation (beware: avoid creating a ledge; Fig 7-11). The transition from interproximal to buccal and lingual can be gently rounded. Some buccal reduction is required with some teeth. This is not usually planned in classic SSC preparation; this is why, if at all, the procedure should be very subtle, protecting the cervical enamel bulge (see Tip 4 below).

Fig 7-12 *(a)* Occlusal view with crown in place. *(b)* Buccal view revealing ischemia immediately after insertion.

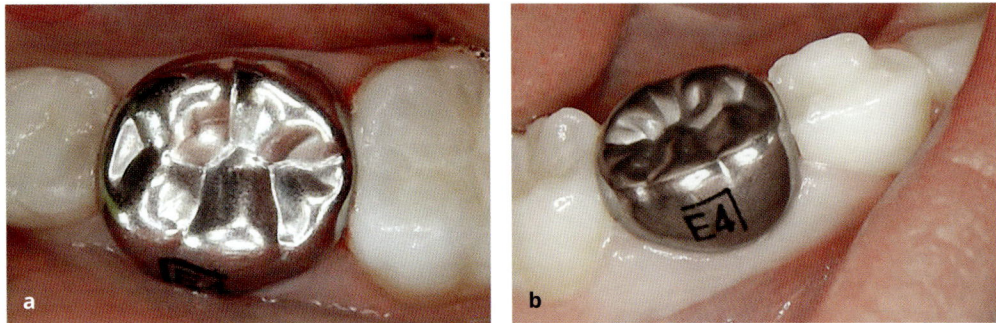

- Then try in the crown, which has to snap over the cervical enamel bulge. The "click effect" is clinically an important sign that the fit is right. The crown can be removed from the primary tooth again using a spatula or a Myrtle blade. The crown must be firmly fixed during the try-in to prevent swallowing or aspiration. It is advisable to have the dental assistant on standby with high-speed suction, ready to suck in the crown if the dentist loses hold of it.

If the crown fits well, it can be cemented with a GIC. Before cementation, a diamond can be used to roughen the intaglio of the crown and thereby increase retention. To insert the crown, either press it down with a finger or ask the child to bite shut with or without a cotton wool roll and thereby push the crown into position. For cementation, the crown should be filled up with enough cement. Any excess cement that leaks out can be wiped away with a swab or cotton wool roll. If the dentist has to work quickly because of limited cooperation and the crown margins lie subgingivally, the excess cement can also be removed with water spray and suction. Clean the interproximal areas with dental floss (dental floss holders are ideal in the primary dentition). Any ischemia that may be visible will disappear a few minutes after crown insertion (Fig 7-12).

The temporary increase in vertical occlusal height that may occur is not a problem in the dynamic child dentition and is compensated by elongation and/or intrusion of the other teeth and usually tolerated by the child without any difficulty. Children will only feel the crown as a foreign body for 1 or 2 days. It is important to communicate the foreign body sensation to the parents and the child. SSC losses are very rare if they fit well. However, children should avoid overly sticky snacks (which they should do anyway for cariogenic reasons). If an SSC comes loose, it can often be recemented in place after cleaning.

TIPS FOR CLASSIC SSC PREPARATION
- **Tip 1:** If a pulpotomy or pulpectomy is performed in the same working step, it is advisable to carry out the occlusal reduction as the first step prior to endodontic treatment. This gives the dentist a much better occlusal view without creating distracting overhangs from cusps.

⟶

- **Tip 2:** If the parents have a problem with the appearance of the crown (children hardly ever have a problem), the open face technique can be used. This involves, usually in a second session, removing the vestibular part of the crown and creating a veneer by means of bonding with a tooth-colored composite. Admittedly the esthetic outcome cannot be compared to a completely tooth-colored crown.
- **Tip 3:** The mandibular first molars are sometimes very wide buccolingually. In such cases, a crown for the opposing primary first molar should be tried.
- **Tip 4:** If migration of the teeth occurs because of severe interproximal caries and hence there is a loss of space, the crown will fit into the mesiodistal width but will be far too narrow in the buccolingual direction. In such cases, slight buccal and lingual preparation and slight bending of the crowns with forceps may become necessary. For example, a Howe plier is well suited for adjusting crowns.

Conclusion for SSCs

For the primary dentition, the prefabricated SSC is a safe, long-term option for restoring primary teeth in highly caries-active children that is not very user- or technique-sensitive. Its only drawback is the esthetic outcome, although the children themselves usually have no problem with these "knight's teeth." Especially with children who do not cooperate as well, the treatment outcome is better than when placing a multilayered adhesive filling. As with any treatment in the primary dentition, the skill of managing the child well during the treatment is necessary more than special expertise. I can only recommend that every colleague "have a go" at this type of restoration. Prefabricated SSCs are often covered by dental insurance and Medicaid.

Colleagues Dobersch-Paulus and Feierabend summarized the most important point as follows in a "plea for the primary tooth crown":

"The plea for child crowns is at the same time a cause that we should champion for children. Is it not among the children's basic rights to receive an acceptable dental restoration? Children are not tiny adults, so they need different treatments. However, the focus of these treatments should be the child, not the parents and not the dentist. Otherwise, an unwarranted significance would be attached to Margolis' words that 'the restoration of carious, fractured or discolored primary anterior teeth [...] is frequently rewarding for dentists because it gives them the certainty of having restored the smile and the self-confidence of a growing child.' The first priority is the child and the child's needs; everything else is of secondary importance."[59–61]

Prefabricated tooth-colored child crowns

There are suppliers of tooth-colored prefabricated child crowns for the anterior and posterior region. These crowns are either made from zirconia or ceramic-modified composite. As the use of these crowns is more difficult and demands greater patient compliance, their use is rather uncommon in general dentistry practices. Much more preparation is required than for SSCs, the preparation margins lie subgingivally, a bleeding-free situation needs to be set up, and, once the tooth has been prepared for a zirconia crown, there is no other restorative option because of the absence of the cervical enamel bulge. The relatively high purchase costs are an added factor. For the sake of completeness, however, this form of restoration is outlined briefly below.

Zirconia crowns

There are now several suppliers of zirconia crowns for children (eg, NuSmile, EZCrowns [Sprig Oral Health Technologies]). What they all have in common is their more complex and necessarily circular preparation because the crowns must be seated on the primary tooth absolutely tension-free. Furthermore, the prefabricated crowns cannot be modified or only to a small extent. Most suppliers therefore offer colored, so-called "try-in crowns," which can be used to establish the right size without contaminating the correct zirconia crown in the mouth during try-in.

As with classic crown preparation, occlusal reduction by as much as 2 mm (depending on the manufacturer's instructions) is followed by circular equigingival preparation (0.8 to 1.5 mm substance removed). The buccal enamel bulge must be completely removed to guarantee tension-free seating. As this lies subgingivally, depending on the child's age, a preparation border up to 2 mm subgingivally may be required. Figure 7-13 clearly shows the greatest challenge posed by preparation.[62]

Once the correct crown has been identified with the aid of try-in crowns, the preparation limit is moved subgingivally. Many crown suppliers offer special preparation kits. The crowns are inserted with self-adhesive resin-based cements (which require a bleeding-free working field), GICs, or resin-modified GICs, depending on manufacturer information. Because the primary teeth have to be prepared subgingivally, hemostasis is an important and yet difficult working step.

The greatest advantage of zirconia crowns is their excellent biocompatibility and more attractive esthetics. The preparation rules are presented in Fig 7-14. Figure 7-15 demonstrates the preparation, hemostasis, and completion of two NuSmile zirconia crowns on the mandibular right primary molars after preceding pulpotomy with mineral trioxide aggregate (MTA), as well as the crowns functioning after 1 year.

Ceramic-modified composite crowns

These tooth-colored crowns made from high-performance acrylic are supplied in four sizes for anterior teeth and six sizes for primary molars and the 6-year molars. The crowns are seated with a dual-setting composite. According to the manufacturer, the crowns can be individualized with cross-cut burs or hard silicone before being seated.

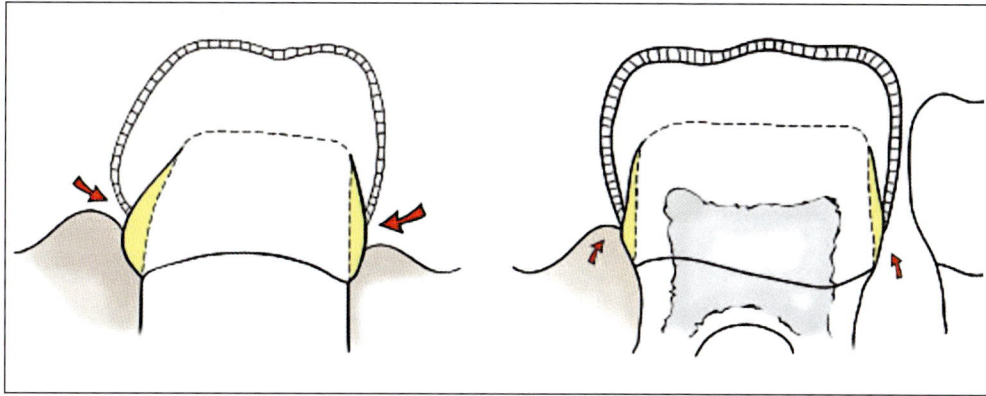

Fig 7-13 Preparation rules for tooth-colored primary molar crowns: While the buccal enamel bulge remains fully preserved with SSCs, with zirconia crowns this area has to be prepared entirely subgingivally so that tension-free seating can be guaranteed. Depending on the position of the cervical enamel bulge, this requires a preparation border lying up to 2 mm subgingivally. (Courtesy of Sprig Oral Health Technologies.[62])

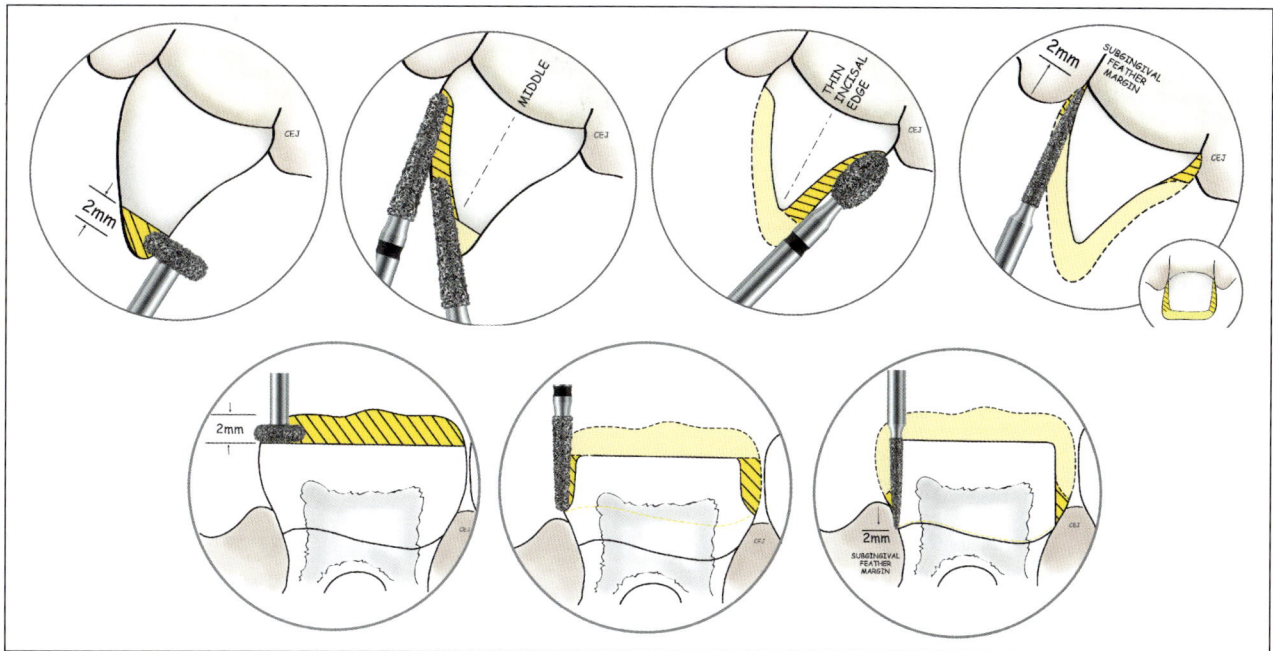

Fig 7-14 Procedure for fabrication of a zirconia crown in the anterior and posterior dentition. (Courtesy of Sprig Oral Health Technologies.[62])

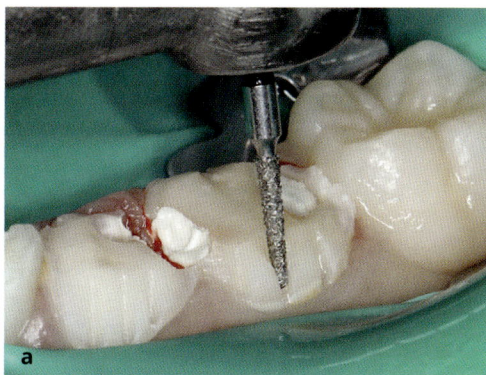

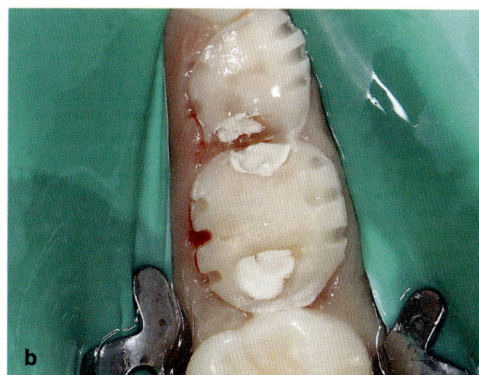

Fig 7-15 (a and b) After carrying out occlusal reduction of approximately 2 mm, depth markings were made buccally and lingually so that circular substance removal during preparation could be controlled more effectively. The amount removed for circumferential preparation is approximately 1 to 1.3 mm.

119

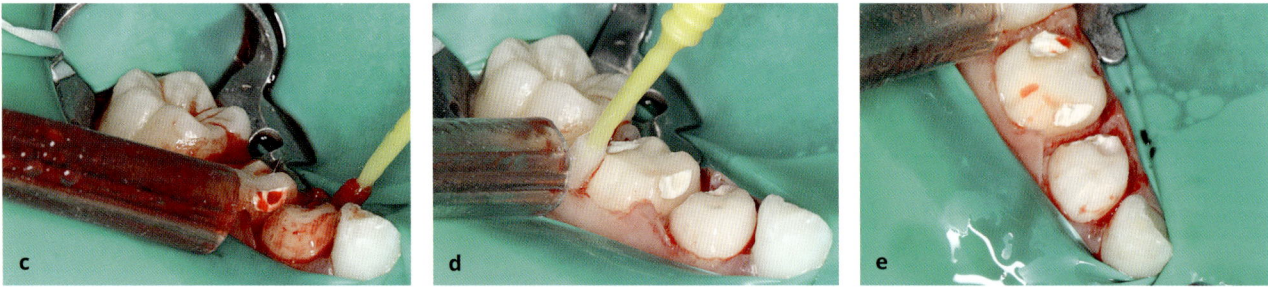

Fig 7-15 *(cont)* *(c and d)* Hemostasis after subgingival preparation. *(e)* Situation before seating of the crowns. *(f and g)* Cementation of the crowns. *(h to j)* Follow-up of the crowns after 1 year. (Courtesy of Dr Jorge Casián Adem.)

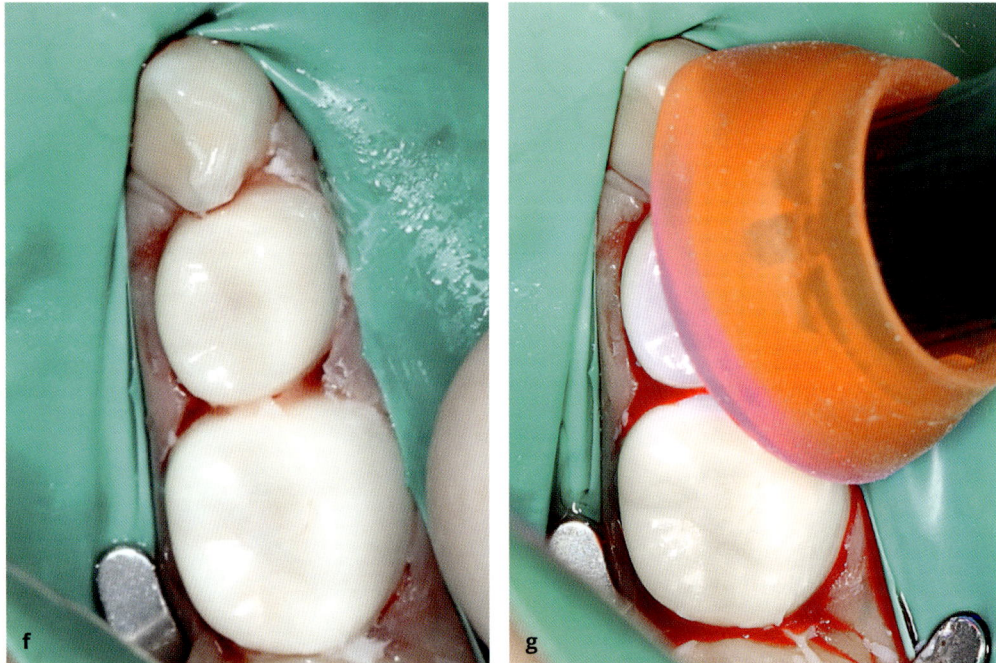

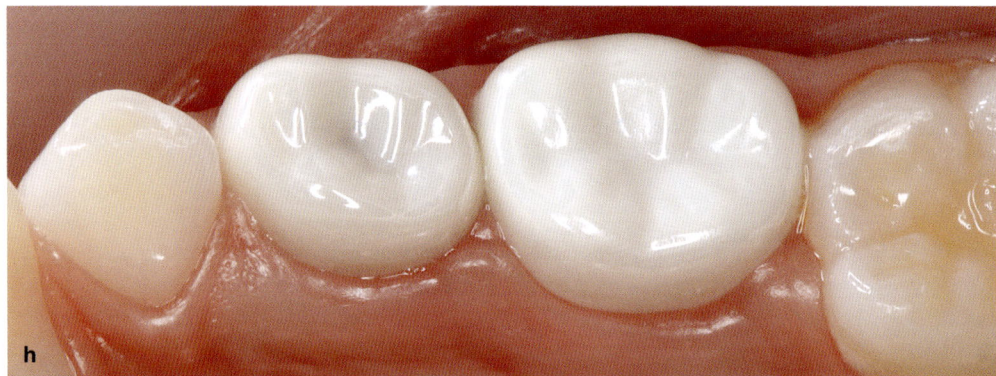

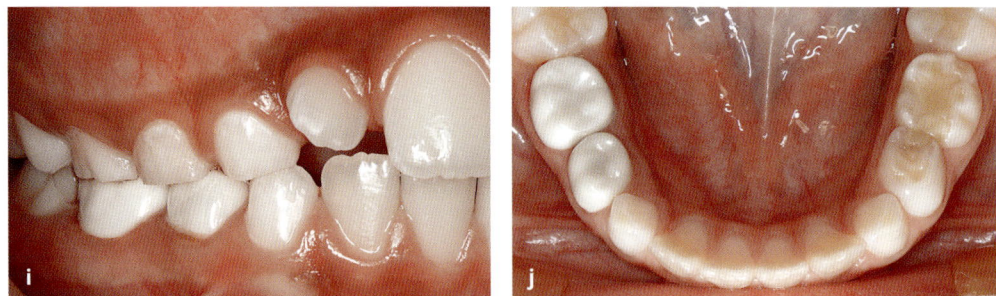

Some grinding even after seating is supposed to be possible. According to the information from the manufacturer, the crowns can also be modified in the mouth with veneer acrylic. As with zirconia crowns, preparation is more extensive than with SSCs because absolutely tension-free seating must be guaranteed. There is still no data for retention rates, abrasion grades, and user-friendliness.

Conclusion for tooth-colored crowns

Even if parents' demand for tooth-colored restorations continues to grow, zirconia crowns or crowns made of high-performance acrylic cannot replace prefabricated SSCs in pediatric dentistry. Especially in general dentistry practices, where there are usually no sedation facilities, routine use of tooth-colored crowns should be viewed critically. The preparation is more complex, the technique is more user-sensitive, and the child's compliance must accordingly be far greater. Extensive studies on long-term stability are still not available because as yet there have been only a few studies on zirconia crowns, for instance. Lauenstein summarizes as follows: "The prefabricated steel crown continues to be an easy to use, reliable and durable treatment option in pediatric dentistry. Their use can be learnt and mastered even by practitioners as yet inexperienced in this field, so that they can help to reduce the significant level of unrestored primary dentitions and ultimately further cut the high prevalence of caries in this area."[54]

Strip (Frasaco) crowns for the anterior teeth

Strip crowns are particularly well suited to the restoration of heavily involved anterior teeth. As a limitation for nonspecialist practices, however, it must be said that the indication for restoring anterior teeth with crowns only applies up to a maximum of 4 years of age and demands good cooperation from the child.[60] As a result, this type of restoration is rather rare in general dentistry practices, but it is outlined briefly here. The range of indications encompasses primary teeth destroyed by caries, traumatically damaged primary teeth, or restoration of mineralization disorders.

Strip crowns are available in different sizes for central and lateral incisors and canines. The crowns for the maxillary lateral incisors can readily be used for the mandibular anterior teeth. The dental hard tissue should be reduced occlusally by about 1.5 mm and proximally by about 1 mm. This reduction usually arises during the course of caries excavation. If the dental hard tissue is intact, the aprismatic enamel layer should be removed labially and palatally.[60]

After caries excavation, select the correct crown and trim to size at the crown margin with scissors. If the tooth has severe caries, a composite core can be prepared prior to crown restoration. Then punch two vents in the corners of the crown with a probe so that excess filling material can escape when pressure is applied. The primary tooth should be pretreated by the acid-etch technique and with an adhesive; if a composite core was necessary, this should be reconditioned. Then fill the crown with a flowable composite or a mixture of packable and flowable composite. Available colors are A1 (can look slightly yellowish in the white primary dentition), Tetric basic white (Ivoclar Vivadent), or what are known as "pedo shades" that reproduce the white, slightly bluish gleam of the primary

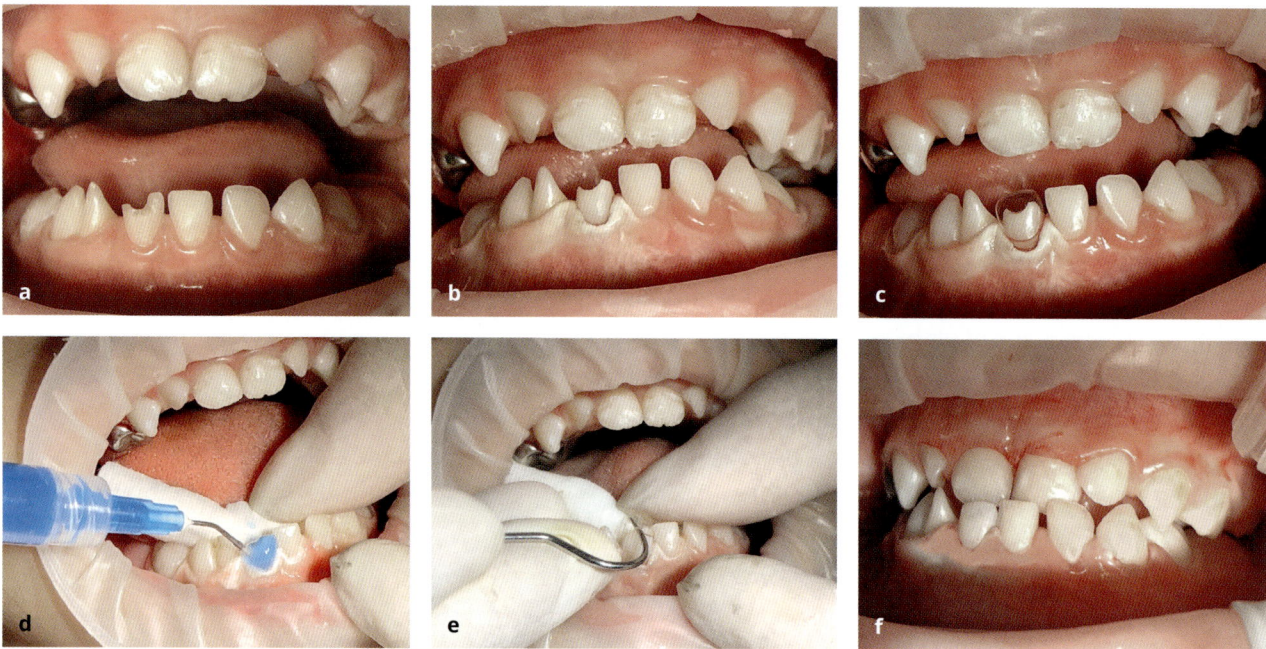

Fig 7-16 Strip crown in the anterior mandible. *(a)* Preoperative condition. *(b)* Preparation and hemostasis using retraction cord. *(c)* Try-in of the Frasaco crown. *(d)* Acid-etch technique under a relative dry field. *(e)* Detaching the crown after setting. *(f)* Condition after finishing. (Courtesy of Dr Nicola Meissner.)

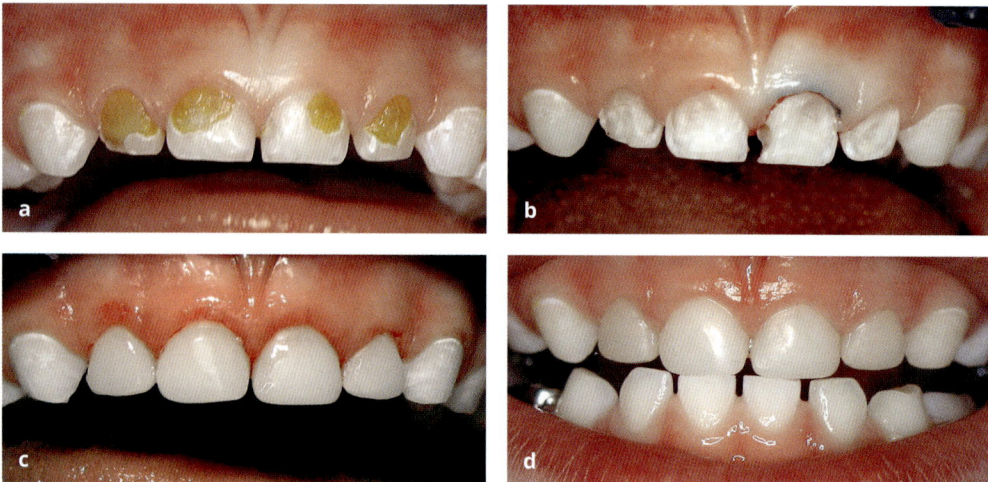

Fig 7-17 Strip crowns in the anterior maxilla. *(a)* Preoperative view. *(b)* Condition after caries excavation. *(c)* Condition after finishing. *(d)* Follow-up with excellent gingival conditions. (Courtesy of Dr Nicola Meissner.)

teeth. Then push the filled crown slowly over the tooth preparation. Remove excess filling material cervically and incisally. Finally, light cure the crown for 20 seconds from each side. After removal of the strip crown form, finish and polish the crown. Palatal adjustment is usually required for the benefit of the occlusion.[60]

Figure 7-16 shows the preparation of a strip crown for a mandibular anterior tooth. Maxillary anterior teeth can also be esthetically reproduced by means of strip crowns. Figure 7-17 show the reconstruction of maxillary primary teeth. Even very heavily involved anterior teeth in advanced ECC can be preserved with the aid of strip crowns after pulpectomy and composite cores (Fig 7-18).

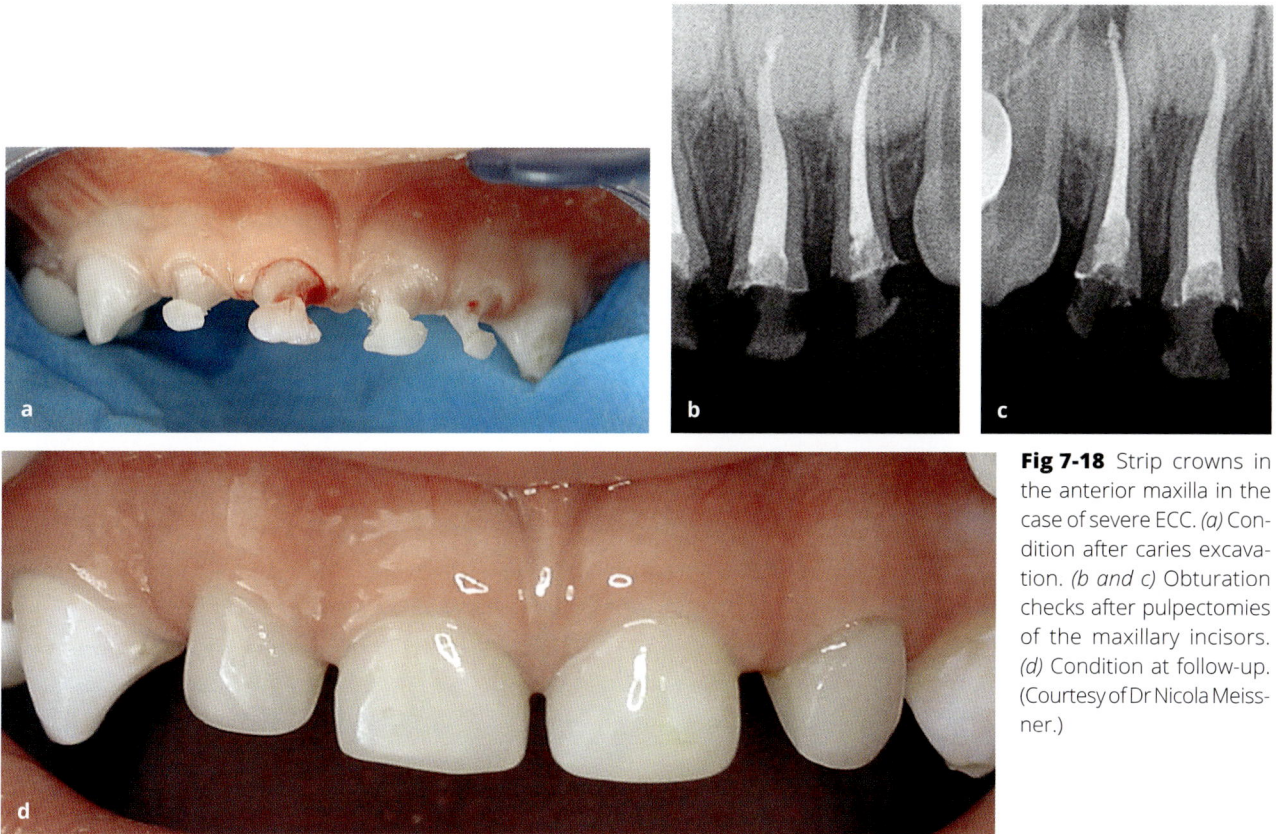

Fig 7-18 Strip crowns in the anterior maxilla in the case of severe ECC. *(a)* Condition after caries excavation. *(b and c)* Obturation checks after pulpectomies of the maxillary incisors. *(d)* Condition at follow-up. (Courtesy of Dr Nicola Meissner.)

BASIC PRINCIPLES OF CARIES AND ENDODONTIC TREATMENT IN CHILDREN

Superficial carious lesions in the primary dentition do not usually pose a particular challenge and can often be well sealed, excavated, and filled or arrested. It is often the cavitated dentin lesions close to the pulp that challenge patients and the dental practitioner. At times the quality of the restoration is very poor, and it is not uncommonly associated with filling losses and pulp necrosis.

Principles of caries treatment and primary tooth endodontics are explained below. There is a discussion of whether measures we successfully apply to the permanent teeth are also indicated for the primary dentition.

Measures for preserving vitality of primary tooth pulp

Indirect capping

These measures are described in the literature either as "caries profunda" therapy or "indirect capping." They are indicated if the defect (caused by trauma or caries) is very close to the pulp but the pulp is still closed. In recent years, there has been an increasing shift away from complete excavation of caries, with priority given to leaving residual caries in place in favor of preserving pulp integrity. Many studies have shown that iatrogenic pulp exposure can thereby be avoided, and the vitality of the primary tooth pulp can be maintained. Depending on the activity of the carious lesion, the residual caries close to the pulp may be either hard on probing and darkly discolored (chronic caries), or the dentin consistency may be leathery (active carious lesion had existed).[36]

Crucially for the success of treatment, regardless of the filling material chosen, the cavity margin must be caries-free to guarantee an absolutely tight restoration. Cavity lining in terms of a calcium hydroxide preparation is not necessary. The single-phase method is preferred to the two-phase method (ie, complete caries excavation in a second session after the formation of tertiary dentin), partly because it is easier to perform in practice. The prognosis is favorable if the thickness of residual dentin over the pulp is 0.5 to 1 mm. If the dentin is thinner and the pulp shows through, the dentist should perform a pulpotomy. In this case, indirect capping is very likely to result in pulp necrosis, often with fistula formation.

Of course, it must be said that the assessment of residual dentin thickness on radiographs and its measurement during caries excavation in the mouth can only be a mere estimate by the dental practitioner. Whether to leave residual caries in place, completely excavate, and/or perform an endodontic measure in the form of a pulpotomy must ultimately be decided afresh with each patient and for every tooth. There will always be successes and failures; it is important to thoroughly weigh the decision and take account of the influencing factors (compliance, defect size, symptoms, etc).

CAUTION ABOUT INDIRECT CAPPING

Pediatric dentists, in particular, often encounter failures of partial caries removal in the primary dentition because the cornerstones of successful caries profunda treatment frequently are not or cannot be achieved in practice. It is also worth bearing in mind that very positive study results in this situation were often obtained in a university setting with a specific patient selection. These circumstances usually cannot be translated directly to general dentistry practices. Of course, leaving residual caries close to the pulp can work provided the following conditions are met:

- The tooth was symptom-free prior to treatment.
- The child is very cooperative so that it is possible to create a sufficiently dry field during filling placement (depending on the nature of the material used).
- The defect in the dental hard tissue is supragingival and does not exceed a class II cavity.
- The cavity margins are absolutely caries-free.

It needs to be stated clearly that this is not the situation with many carious lesions in the primary dentition, and it is difficult to obtain a reliable pain history for a child. If the indication is correct, indirect capping will achieve better long-term results than pulpotomy.[63] With regard to success rates (no

→

pain, inflammation, interradicular radiolucencies, or fistulae), the treatment method performs very well if a tight seal is achieved (96% in a 3-year observation period).[64]

It should be noted that fillings under which residual caries was left in place need to be checked regularly and repaired or renewed more frequently.[65]

Before opting for indirect capping, dentists should realistically assess their own skills dependent on the patient's compliance. Especially for children with limited cooperation, when it might be difficult to guarantee a bacterially tight seal over the filling, the Hall technique (see previous section) may prove a better choice in terms of preserving the vitality of the primary tooth. When children are very cooperative, more cautious excavation can certainly be done. If there is evidence of reversible pulpitis (stimulus-dependent pains; no constant and/or spontaneous pain), in some circumstances a pulpotomy followed by crown restoration may be the safer treatment pathway. For lesions where the pulp shows through, pulpotomy has the better prognosis in the author's experience.

Here again it is true that there are several possible approaches, but not every option is right for every patient, and you will not always be successful. Thorough education of the parents and careful consideration of all the accompanying factors play a significant role.

Direct capping

Direct capping is hardly ever indicated in the primary dentition, and this treatment is problematic in several respects. In many countries direct capping is actually contraindicated for the primary molar region.[66] In the course of caries removal, the author considers this method to be unsuitable for several reasons. First, the dentist cannot say with certainty that the dentin at the site of exposure was absolutely free of caries. Second, microbial transmission into the exposed pulp by the dentist cannot be ruled out. And third, the repair capacity of the exposed primary tooth pulp is very poor. As we know that a residual dentin thickness of less than 0.5 mm can be prognostically judged highly unfavorable for preserving vital pulp (see "Indirect capping"), the method of direct capping in caries treatment is more than questionable for that reason. The risk of the primary tooth pulp being infected, at least in the coronal portion, is too high. If a pulpotomy is already recommended in the case of indirect capping where the residual dentin thickness is less than 0.5 mm because the outcome is better, in the author's opinion there are justifiable doubts about the success of any direct pulp capping in the process of caries removal.

In case of trauma, assuming a primarily healthy pulp, the question arises of whether any contamination has taken place between the time of the trauma and the visit to the dentist. Once again, the advice is likely to be pulpotomy. However, especially anterior dental trauma usually occurs in the primary dentition at an age when cooperation for pulpotomy does not exist in very many patients or physiologic root resorption has already advanced so far that extraction is more worth considering for a complicated coronal fracture.

For direct capping in caries-free dentin, MTA or an aqueous calcium hydroxide preparation is applied to the "non-bleeding exposed site," and the tooth is provided with a tight restoration.[36]

In conclusion, direct capping in the primary dentition during caries removal is rather questionable and additionally has a very narrow range of indications. As ever, the prevailing circumstances obviously need to be taken into consideration. If the child is very cooperative and can provide reliable information about previous pain symptoms, if a primary anterior tooth is affected, and, in case of doubt, the child will readily accept further treatment, direct capping can be performed if the indication is correct. If not, a pulpotomy (possibly followed by crown restoration) will in most cases provide a more stable outcome in the long term. Correct patient selection (no continuous and/or spontaneous pain, no interradicular radiolucency, bleeding that is easy to stop and light red in color, root is no more than one-third resorbed) is again a prerequisite. For primary molars, Heinrich-Weltzien and Kühnisch (2007) give the following assessment of direct capping: "As direct capping is recommended solely on the basis of clinical experience and expert opinions, the level of evidence is only classed as grade C for primary molars. [...] The form of treatment of direct capping must be viewed critically because of the high failure rate for primary teeth."[66]

Pulpotomy (vital amputation)

Many dentists are wary of performing endodontic treatments in the primary dentition. The next section is intended to bring pulpotomy into general dentistry practice as a simple and very promising treatment method, to instill confidence in its application, and thereby expand dentists' range of treatments with an important pediatric dentistry measure. Pulpotomy is the most commonly performed endodontic treatment in the primary dentition.

Pulpotomy is a vitality-preserving measure. Assuming the indication has been properly established and the tooth is ideally restored with a crown after pulpotomy, success rates of 80% to 90% are given for this treatment method over a 2-year observation period.[36] It offers several advantages to both dental practitioner and child: only one session, good prospects of success and retention rates, and speedy treatment. If the tooth in question still has enough residual enamel and is expected to remain in the mouth for 2 years or less, a tight filling can be placed after pulpotomy.[63] For extensive defects and if the tooth will be in the mouth for longer, subsequent crown restoration is closely associated with treatment success.

The correct indication should always be established before pulpotomy. The greatest source of error lies in performing the treatment outside of the indications, which can result in fistulae, pain, or premature tooth loss. Pulpotomy is possible provided that the following conditions are met:

• There is no constant or nocturnal pain because that suggests irreversible pulpitis. In this case, an attempt to preserve vitality should be abandoned and priority given to pulpectomy or extraction. Brief stimulus-dependent pains, which are close timewise to attendance at the dental office, are no obstacle to pulpotomy because it may be assumed that only the coronal part of the pulp is affected by pulpitis.

- Root resorption is no more advanced than one-third.
- No interradicular radiolucency can be seen on radiographs.
- No fistula is present.
- The tooth will still exhibit enough dental hard tissue after pulpotomy for it to be tightly sealed. This is almost always possible, at least with a prefabricated SSC.
- Bleeding from the radicular portion of the pulp is arrested after 30 seconds. If this is not the case, it suggests pulpitis that is no longer confined to the coronal pulp.

If these criteria are met, a pulpotomy can be performed. If the pulp in the carious dentin is exposed in the course of caries excavation, the pulp roof can be removed immediately with a diamond. Under water cooling, the coronal pulp is then removed with a no. 4 or 6 round bur or diamond burs. For the latter, preference should be given to those with non-diamond–coated tips to avoid damage to the pulp base. It is advisable to remove the pulp at the upper canal entry in a punctate fashion. Iron(III) sulfate is suitable for hemostasis. The preparation (eg, Astringedent, Ultradent) leads to vessel sealing without the formation of a coagulum, which is crucial to successful development of a hard tissue bridge.[66] Standard saline solution also works very well. Zinc oxide eugenol cement with resin molecules (eg, IRM, Dentsply) or MTA are suitable for coverage, the latter being the most biocompatible but also the most expensive option. Calcium hydroxide performed less well in long-term studies[67] but is preferred in Scandinavian countries.

If the bleeding cannot be stopped within half a minute after application of 15.5% iron(III) sulfate solution (a maximum of one repeated attempt can be made) or after 3 minutes when just using standard saline solution, this suggests inflammation of the pulp beyond the upper third. If so, the tooth should either be extracted immediately or a pulpectomy should be performed.[36]

> **TIP FOR PULPOTOMY**
>
> If the tooth is to be restored with an SSC after a planned pulpotomy, it is advisable to start with the occlusal reduction first after anesthesia, hence the first step of SSC preparation. This allows far better visualization of the pulp cavity. It is just as well to finish the complete crown preparation first, do the pulpotomy afterward, and then try in the steel crowns while hemostasis is in progress. Figure 7-19 shows the sequence of a pulpotomy with MTA and subsequent cementation of an SSC.

In conclusion, the following are the most important criteria for successful pulpotomy: correct patient selection, hemostasis without leaving a blood clot, the right wound dressing (MTA or IRM), and a tight restoration. In those circumstances, the success rate for this form of treatment is very high. As enough residual enamel for a tight adhesive filling and very good cooperation are required, the SSC is the recommended form of restoration

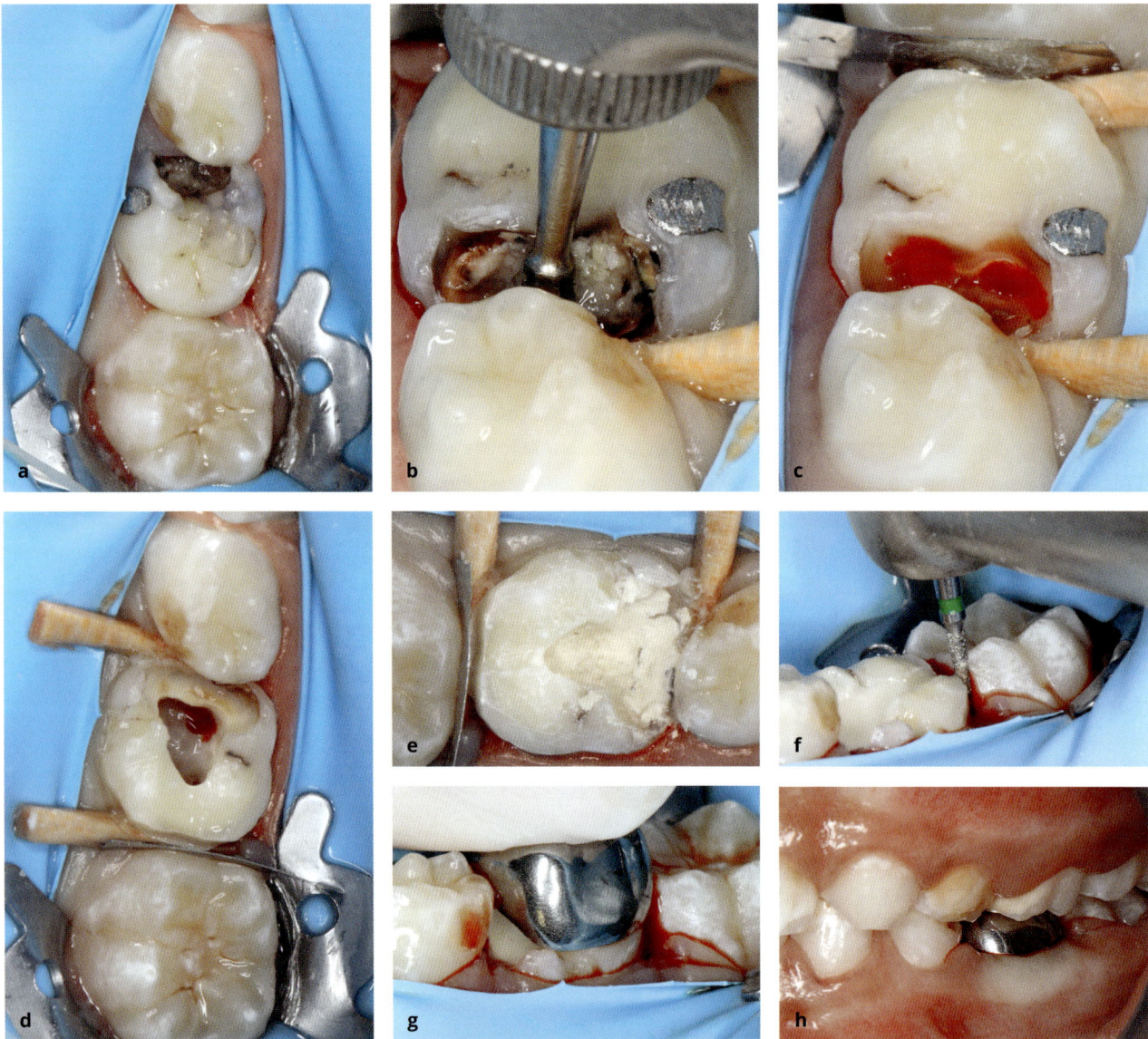

Fig 7-19 Pulpotomy and restoration with an SSC in the primary dentition. *(a)* Preoperative view of the mandibular primary second molar. *(b)* Caries removal. *(c)* Pulp exposure. *(d)* View into the pulp cavity. *(e)* Application of MTA. *(f)* Interproximal separation in the course of SSC preparation. *(g)* Try-in of the SSC. *(h)* Seated SSC and buccal ischemia immediately after insertion. *(i)* Seated SSC. *(j)* Radiograph after completed pulpotomy. Interproximal cement residues are still visible mesially and have to be removed. (Courtesy of Dr Jorge Casián Adem.)

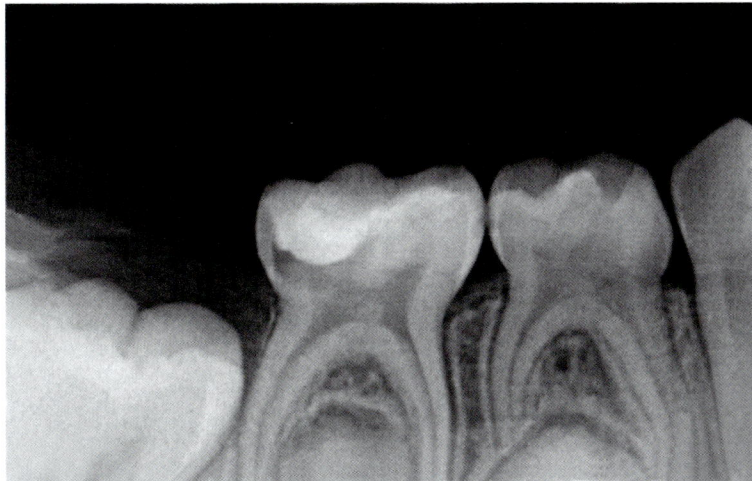

Fig 7-20 Indication for pulpectomy at the mandibular primary second molar. The child is 4 years old and has already had frequent nocturnal toothache, which has been treated with ibuprofen by the mother; there is no interradicular radiolucency. The aim is tooth preservation until the permanent 6-year molar erupts.

for teeth commonly affected by deep interproximal defects. If wound closure is to be performed with a zinc oxide eugenol preparation, a cavity lining (eg, GIC) must be placed if an adhesive filling is planned because of the plasticizer function.

Endodontics in primary teeth: Pulpectomy

Pulpectomy, or root canal treatment of the primary tooth, is certainly of minor significance in general dentistry practice. Fistulating teeth or primary teeth with manifest inflammation must be extracted and not undergo pulpectomy. A reasonable indication for pulpectomy might exist in the case of irreversible pulpitis (spontaneous pain not dependent on stimulus, frequent nocturnal pain) affecting the primary second molars while the permanent first molars have not yet erupted. In this situation, it can be very difficult to prepare a space maintainer distally (eg, a fixed space maintainer with distal shoe) if the primary second molar is extracted. Hence there is a risk that the gap will be narrowed by the permanent first molar. An attempt to preserve the tooth may thus be advisable in this case, provided that the child is very cooperative, the primary tooth is not entirely destroyed and can subsequently be conservatively restored, and advanced inflammation is not present (Fig 7-20).

Even the indication for pulpectomy of the primary anterior teeth is limited: It is only indicated up to the age of 4 years. Before that, children are rarely cooperative enough to make a pulpectomy feasible in standard treatment, and after that physiologic resorption commences. For primary molars, pulpectomy is only indicated up to the age of 8 or 9 years. The prognosis of pulpectomy is better for primary anterior teeth than for molars.[36] The following paragraphs condense primary tooth pulpectomy into essential key points for general dentistry practice.

A radiograph should be taken before pulpectomy in order to exclude advanced interradicular inflammation. The root growth of the primary tooth must be completed, but there must not yet be any discernible signs of physiologic resorption.[36] The author considers the use of a rubber dam for pulpectomy as absolutely essential and would not

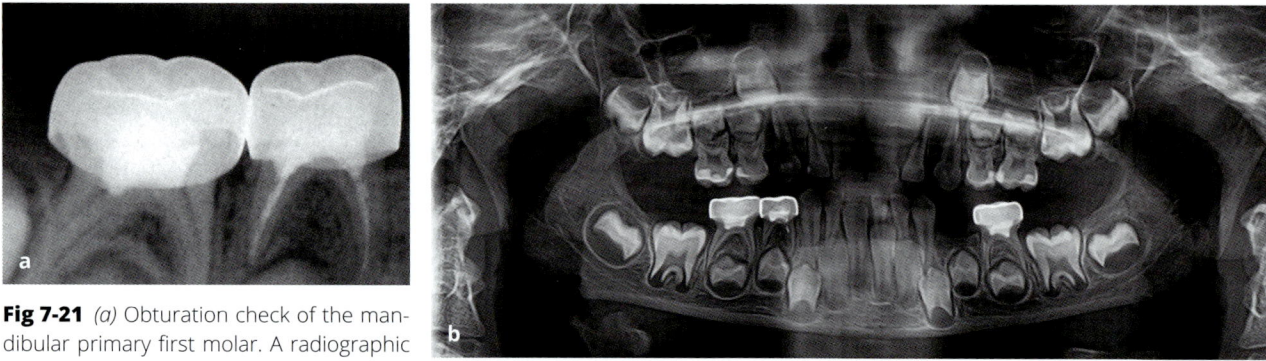

Fig 7-21 (a) Obturation check of the mandibular primary first molar. A radiographic obturation check is advisable so that correct filling of the pulpectomy can be verified. The primary second molar was treated by pulpotomy. Both teeth were fitted with SSCs. (b) Almost fully resorbed root filling observed on the radiographic check after 2 years. The root filling material was Vitapex.

perform a pulpectomy if the child is not compliant enough. After anesthesia the pulp roof is taken off, the pulp is completely removed, and preparation is started. Pulpectomy of a primary tooth is a challenge for both child and dentist. It can occasionally be difficult to extirpate or even do preparation for a terminal primary molar when there is minimal mouth opening. While preparation is easier for primary anterior teeth, greater importance is attached to disinfection with irrigating solutions in the case of primary molars. Sodium hypochlorite (NaOCl, 1% to 2%) and additionally 2% CHX are recommended as irrigating solutions. If both are used, neutralizing physiologic saline must be applied in between to prevent complex formation. Preparation of the root canals should only be done with instruments above ISO size 20 in order to prevent overinstrumentation.[68] Preparation length should be controlled with electrometric or radiographic measures, but the author finds the latter particularly difficult in practice and not easily workable.

Anyone who lacks the facility for electrometric probing can follow the advice in the publication by Heinrich-Weltzien and Kühnisch in the textbook by Splieth from 2002. They measured the mean root lengths and variances for primary anterior teeth and primary molars. The approximate preparation lengths can be deduced from these figures. The mean root lengths ranged from 13 to 16 mm for primary molars, measured at the appropriate cusps.[69] The aim is to prepare up to 2 mm before the apex. By implication this means that an acceptable result can be achieved with a working length of 11 to 12 mm. If, before pulpectomy, the tooth is shortened occlusally by 2 mm for the subsequent crown restoration, the working length must be additionally reduced by this amount.[34]

Only fully resorbable materials, for example iodoform pastes (Vitapex), an aqueous calcium hydroxide preparation, or calcium salicylate-based sealer, should be considered as root filling materials.[36] Vitapex, for instance, is actually available in a small trial pack, which is ideal especially for the general dentistry practice. It is simple to use and is applied using a thin cannula. To ensure the material can be applied properly, up to ISO size 30/35 should be used for preparation. Furthermore, adequate disinfection with irrigating solutions should be guaranteed. It should be noted that these filling materials resorb relatively quickly and may no longer be radiographically visible after a certain amount of time (Fig 7-21). Provided the tooth is comfortable and symptom-free, there is no reason for extraction. The best coronal restoration of the teeth is undoubtedly with crowns.

SURGICAL INTERVENTIONS

Extractions in the primary dentition, incision of the lingual and labial frena, and possibly surgical interventions for abscesses are relevant to practitioners working in general dentistry. Extraction of permanent teeth will not be described here because it is a regular feature of general dentistry practice.

Extraction of primary teeth

Fistulating teeth, primary teeth that are severely loosened after trauma or have already undergone considerable pathologic resorption (eg, undermining resorption of the primary second molars by the permanent first molars), or ankylosed primary teeth must be extracted. A radiograph should be taken prior to extraction, provided physiologically loosened primary teeth are not involved.

Children should be prepared in a child-appropriate way for the noises or sensations to be expected. It can help to give children a pictorial explanation of what will happen: "Today we're going to swing your tooth out. Have you ever swung really high in the playground? So high that your tummy feels a bit funny? Well, when I swing your tooth today, you might feel the swinging a little bit."

In principle, we try to pass all the instruments we need under the child's headrest. Forceps for primary teeth are small and can easily disappear in the dentist's hand.

After anesthesia, detach the marginal gingiva with a narrow Bein elevator. In the mixed dentition, it is important to ensure that insertion of an elevator does not loosen adjacent permanent teeth that have not yet completed their root growth. In this case, working with an elevator should be completely avoided.[29] Using the appropriate primary tooth forceps, loosen the tooth in the buccolingual direction and remove it. Primary anterior teeth can be extracted by means of rotating movements. They must not be luxated in the direction of the tooth germ (hence dislodging the primary tooth crown labially). The delicate root apices of primary molars sometimes fracture, which is evident during luxation as a quiet cracking sound. If the primary tooth was infected, carefully remove the root remnants (beware of the tooth germ). If this is primarily a healthy and vital primary tooth, small fragments can be left in place. They are either resorbed or work their way to the surface a little later and can easily be removed with tweezers. Apical curettage is not done for primary tooth extraction because it might damage the tooth germ.

It is important to explain the effect of the anesthetic to children and parents so that bite injuries can be avoided. Such injuries are less common after the use of intraligamentary anesthesia systems.

> **IS A SPACE MAINTAINER ALWAYS NECESSARY?**
> If a primary tooth had to be removed early, hence at least 1 year before physiologic exfoliation, recall should be arranged after a short interval to monitor mesialization of the 6-year molar after loss of the primary second molar and to

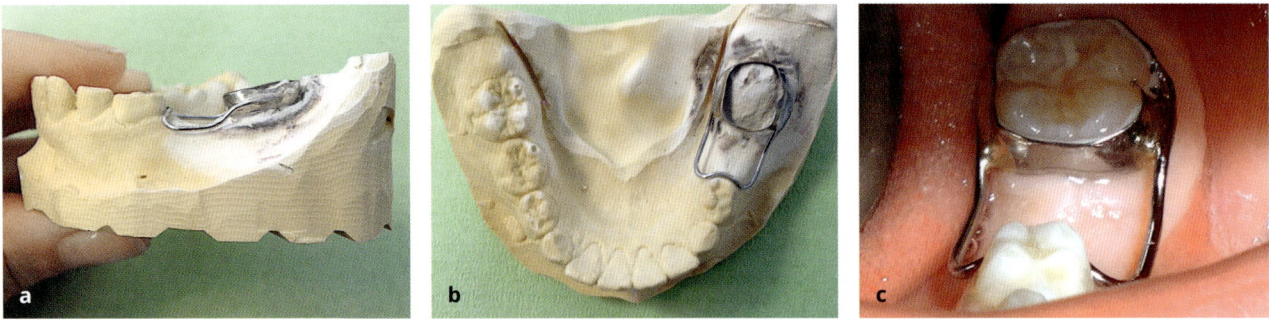

Fig 7-22 *(a to c)* Individual, fixed space maintainer fabricated in the laboratory and affixed in the mouth.

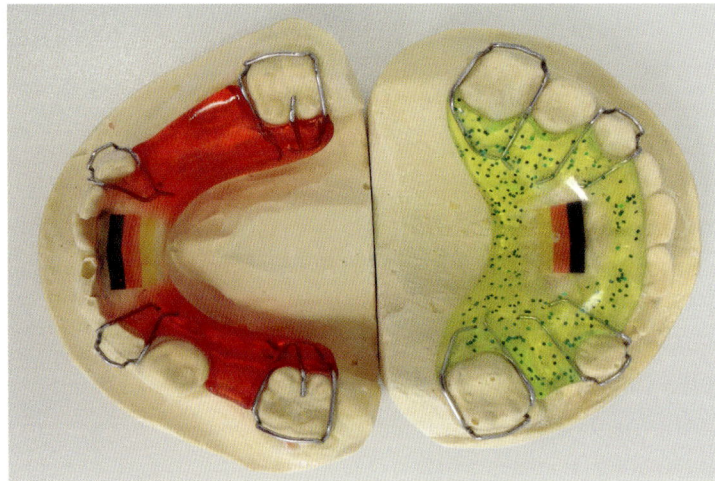

Fig 7-23 Removable space maintainer for the maxillary and mandibular arches.

check the associated narrowing of the gap. Especially if children lose primary molars before eruption of the permanent first molars in the relevant quadrants, there is a risk of gap narrowing in the posterior dentition. Premature loss of primary anterior teeth is more of an esthetic and phonetic problem. Gap narrowing is not to be feared in this case. However, a prosthesis may become necessary from the speech therapy point of view. There are small removable prostheses for children or even fixed appliances where molar bands are cemented around the primary second molars and the primary anterior teeth being replaced are fixed to a wire running palatally.

In the case of reliable patients and children whose permanent first molars stably occlude, watchful waiting can first be adopted and the resulting gap measured regularly. After extraction, we check at the following intervals: 1 week, 4 weeks, 3 months, and 6 months. If gap narrowing of 1 mm or more is observed in the first half-year after extraction, a space maintainer must be prepared.[70]

Removable spacers or fixed spacers can be used for this purpose. Figure 7-22 shows a customized, fixed space maintainer fabricated in the laboratory. Figure 7-23 shows removable spacers.

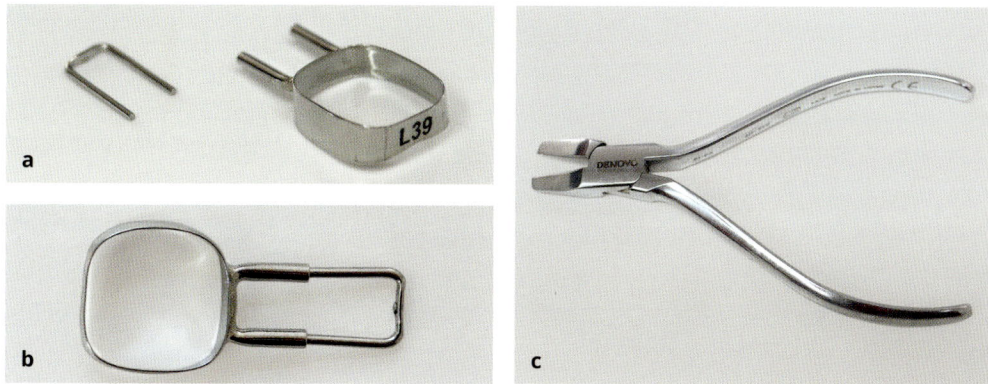

Fig 7-24 *(a to c)* The Denovo space maintainer system. (Courtesy of Claudia Lippold.)

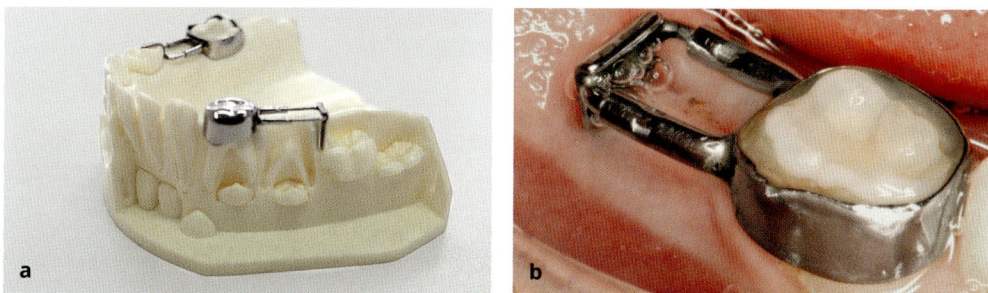

Fig 7-25 *(a)* Denovo space maintainer with distal shoe on the cast. (Courtesy of Claudia Lippold.) *(b)* Denovo space maintainer with distal shoe in situ. (Courtesy of Dr Silvia Träupmann.)

Among fixed spacers there is also the possibility of chairside fabrication. The advantage of the Denovo system is that fixed spacers can be fabricated immediately without taking an impression. This involves selecting an appropriate molar band and a second metal part, which is pushed into the tube fixed to the molar band to the appropriate length and is crimped with special pliers (Fig 7-24). The relatively high purchase costs of the set are rather off-putting for general dentists who might not fabricate many fixed space maintainers.

Alternatively, the teeth in question can be measured beforehand using dental floss and the molar bands ordered individually. Another alternative is provided by laboratory-fabricated, individualized fixed space maintainers, but these do require impression-taking. Equally you may consult specialist colleagues or orthodontists you trust. Fixed space maintainers are contraindicated for gaps beyond two primary molars and multiple gaps that need to be spanned. Unlike removable space maintainers, however, they have the advantage of being totally unreliant on the compliance of children (and parents).

A terminal space maintainer for loss of the primary second molar before eruption of the permanent first molar is a special case. Denovo again provides a solution. For this purpose, a molar band is cemented to the primary first molar, which distally has a metal part called a *distal shoe* (Fig 7-25). Fixed space maintainers can be cemented with phosphate cement or GIC. Roughening the inside of the molar band beforehand with a diamond is advisable.

Both types of space maintainer require regular recall to make sure that eruption of the permanent tooth is not prevented.

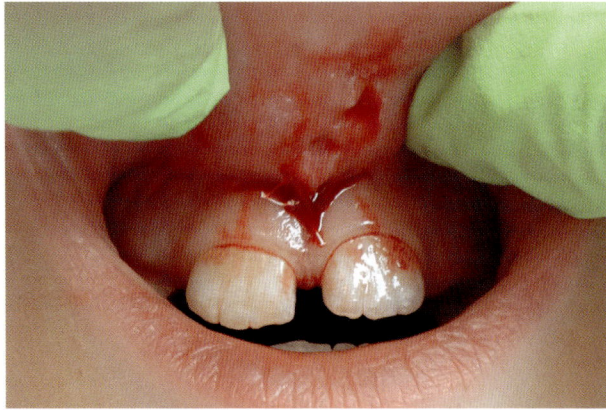

Fig 7-26 Single-knot suture after frenectomy by means of V-Y plasty.

Labial frenum

First it must be stated that preventive frenectomy is not indicated in the primary dentition. A large number of (small) children have a deeply attaching labial frenum in the maxilla without it posing any problem. This will often grow out with increasing age. The only exception is when a labial frenum attaching too deeply proves to be an obstacle to feeding in a newborn baby. This can happen if the frenum is so tight that the top lip is too rigid to allow the baby to reliably latch onto the breast or bottle; ie, the upper lip cannot be folded outward. Admittedly, a labial frenum is only rarely an obstacle to feeding, and, if it is, it will frequently be associated with an overly tight lingual frenum. The latter has a far greater influence on successful feeding.

In all other cases, corrective surgery is not indicated until eruption of the permanent maxillary lateral incisors at the age of 8 to 9 years,[29] or according to other authors not until the permanent maxillary canines erupt.[71] The advantage is that children are far more manageable at this age, and a frenectomy can then be performed far more easily. The procedure is indicated if the incisive papilla becomes ischemic (blanching) when the upper lip is lifted and if there is a midline diastema. At this age and in these cases, there is no point in simply excising the labial frenum with scissors or laser under anesthesia and avoiding the ligamentous apparatus. A V-Y plasty is a simple, extremely suitable method: After surface anesthesia followed by local anesthesia, hold back the top lip while tightening the frenum, then make a V-shaped incision to the labial frenum with a scalpel while sparing the periosteum (the wide base of the "V" lies in the vestibulum, and the pointing top lies in the direction of the teeth). This creates a small, triangular mucosal flap that is detached from the periosteum with a small raspatory and can be advanced upward into the vestibulum. Muscle tracts in the region of the labial frenum are sectioned.[72] If the tissue is completely separated, the decrease in tensile stress when retracting the top lip is noticed immediately. The incision is then closed with a single-knot at the base of the "V" (producing a "Y"). Using resorbable suture material means that the stitch does not have to be removed 5 or 7 days later (Fig 7-26). The lower part of the incision (the downward stroke of the "Y") can be left to secondary healing. This type of dissection can, of course, be done by laser as well.

In 2013, Viergutz and Hetzer described frenectomy according to Eismann: While retracting the upper lip, excise the labial frenum, cut around it in a V-shape, and finally completely remove the soft tissue including periosteum using a sharp spoon. For a labial frenum that also radiates deeply palatally, the same procedure should be followed palatally while sparing the incisive papilla. This produces an "hourglass-shaped" incision.[29]

Lingual frenum

The prevalence of an overly short lingual frenum in newborn infants ranges from 4% to 10% in the literature, a variation caused not least by the lack of standardized diagnostics and classification. In fact, more babies may well be affected.[73] A common finding is a whitish-looking, poorly perfused cord of connective tissue, which fixes the tongue to the floor of the mouth or prevents the middle portion of the tongue from being moved to the palate. In the literature an anatomical distinction is often made between anterior and posterior lingual frena. In the case of the anterior lingual frenum, the connective tissue cord inserts almost entirely at the tip of the tongue and gives the tongue a typical heart shape when attempting to lift it. The posterior lingual frenum is far more difficult to diagnose because the typical cord of connective tissue is absent in many cases, but the dorsum of the tongue still cannot be lifted.[74] The consequences of an excessively tight lingual frenum, apart from possible myofunctional impairments, are faulty jaw development and phonation disorders, especially considerable difficulties in feeding. The children often gain weight poorly, cry a lot, swallow air while drinking, choke, suffer from stomachaches, and are inconsistent in taking breast milk. Mothers suffer from sore nipples, painful engorgement, and ultimately a decreased amount of milk. As a result, they often give up breastfeeding quickly. Furthermore, an untreated tongue-tie can have far-reaching consequences in later child development (see chapter 5 on myofunctional development).

Many midwives and lactation consultants are aware of this problem but often cannot find dental colleagues who will undertake this uncomplicated procedure. In many hospitals the lingual frenum is checked immediately after childbirth and excised if necessary, but unfortunately this does not happen in all hospitals. Some pediatricians will also perform the procedure. Of course, time and again there are critical voices claiming that too short a lingual frenum is not an impediment and "after all, we used to just leave it alone." It may be that the problem was less obvious in the past, for which there are several reasons. First, excessively tight lingual frena would immediately be excised early by a midwife immediately after birth and could not cause any problems. Second, far more women breastfeed now than used to, which means that an overly tight lingual frenum is more likely to cause discomfort for mother and child than is the case when babies are bottle-fed. Another reason why too tight a lingual frenum is more likely to cause problems today is the fact that nursing difficulties frequently result from several different factors. Increasing intervention during childbirth by means of infusions, oxytocin administration, caesarean section, induced labor, epidurals, and analgesia create a number of potential interfering factors in the natural hormonal cascade and can cause changes in mothers that will encourage breastfeeding difficulties (eg, decreasing endogenous oxytocin levels, swollen nipples and areolae, separation of mother and child).[75] This means that, if a mother has favorable anatomical conditions, for instance, has enough milk, and was able to put her child to the breast immediately after birth, the baby may possibly compensate for a lingual frenum that is too short and breastfeed without discomfort. There are also cases, however, where several confounding factors come together and the babies are unable to latch on properly even with minimal restriction of the lingual frenum. To put it another way, not every short lingual frenum needs to be excised in a generalized way. Lingual frenectomy should be performed depending on whether symptoms exist that justify the procedure being carried out.

In the best-case scenario, parents will attend with a baby a few days or weeks old on the recommendation of their pediatrician. Then the "Leipzig protocol" of Dr Springer[76] can be performed to excise the lingual frenum. Even though the procedure is virtually painless and bleeding-free, it is a stressful situation for baby and parents. Good planning and preparation will reduce the unpleasantness for all concerned. It is beneficial if the infant is breastfed immediately before and after the operation. That partly helps to calm the infant and relieve any pain. At the same time it serves the purpose of diagnostics, which consist of three parts: seeing, feeling, and talking. A good light source should be available for visual assessment of the following: To where does the lingual frenum extend? When the child cries, does the tongue form a heart shape? Does the middle part of the tongue touch the palate or only the side areas? In addition, it is important to feel under the baby's tongue with the index fingers, moving the lingual frenum from side to side and moving the tongue upward in order to detect any movement restrictions that are not visible. Finally, history-taking also plays a key role (Is the baby gaining weight satisfactorily? Does the mother experience pain when breastfeeding? Is milk being supplemented with formula?). If the mother breastfeeds while the history is being taken, it is possible to observe at the same time whether the baby is latching on properly and taking milk from all relevant parts of the breast. If the decision is to excise after the diagnostic assessment, there are various options: excision by scalpel, laser, electrotome, or scissors. No option is preferable to any other because success depends solely on the dentist excising all the necessary tissue parts.[74] Excision by laser offers the advantage of hemostasis, but it takes longer in preparation and requires far more technical equipment.[75] Furthermore, the necessary eye protection must obviously be guaranteed for the infant as well. Excision using scissors or scalpel takes just a few seconds. The dentist must have the following ready:

- If appropriate, 20% glucose solution for pain relief and as a mouth-opener.
- Scissors slightly rounded at the tip, scalpel, electrotome, or laser (in the latter case, protective goggles as well).
- A lingual frenum spatula or a wooden spatula from which a V-shape has been cut out on one side (base of the V lies at the end of the spatula). This can be pushed under the tongue so that it can be fixed to the palate and the frenum can thus be tightened.

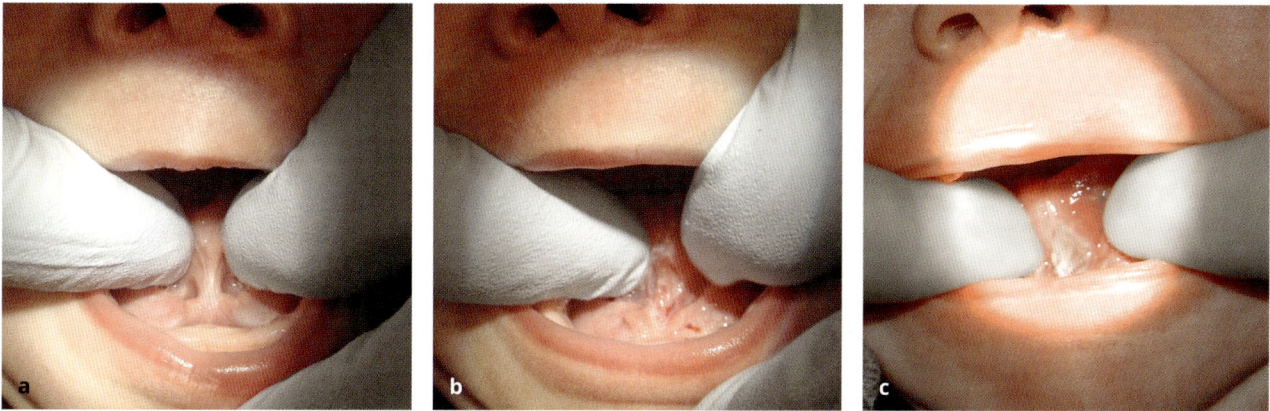

Fig 7-27 Surgical correction of a short lingual frenum. *(a)* Preoperative view. *(b)* Situation immediately after excision. The rhomboid shape of the wound can be seen. *(c)* Situation 1 week after the procedure. (Courtesy of Dr Bobby Ghaheri.)

It is also helpful if the parents swaddle the baby before the treatment, in other words wrapping the baby firmly in a blanket or similar. This makes sure the arms are securely fixed. The nurse holds the baby's head and presses the chin down with her thumb in order to bring about or ensure mouth opening. The tongue is held up with the lingual frenum spatula or modified wooden spatula, and the frenum is excised with a stroke of the scissors. Newman describes his technique as follows: "I use scissors to make a snip at 90 degrees to the edge of the frenulum and cut no more than 1 or 2 mm and then use the index finger of my left hand to push on the cut so that it tears, in the same way as one cuts cloth. When the tongue-tie has been fully released, one sees only a diamond-shaped wound where the frenulum once was." This method causes only minimal bleeding. After excision, the child can be immediately put to the mother's breast.[76] Local anesthesia can be dispensed with, especially when using scissors or scalpel, because babies can be soothed immediately at their mother's breast and only then is it possible to know whether the child is subsequently breastfeeding better and the procedure has been successful. If the sublingual area has been anesthetized, the baby will not be able to latch on properly. Topical anesthesia like lidocaine gel can be used. Figure 7-27 shows a typical preoperative situation of a posterior lingual frenum, the condition immediately after excision, and wound healing after 1 week.

If older children present with this problem, the short frenum cannot be stretched by speech therapy exercises, and if the excessively short lingual frenum causes disorders, it can be excised under local anesthesia. If it radiates between the mandibular anterior teeth, the area can be dissected and the frenum removed in the same way as the procedure for the labial frenum. Once again, laser can be used for this purpose. Some authors recommend stretching exercises after excision in order to prevent reattachment,[73] while other authors doubt the usefulness of these exercises.[75]

The author is of the opinion that an individual decision can certainly be considered depending on the characteristics of the frenum, the time of cutting, and the way the baby is fed. If active wound management (AWM) is recommended, the author thinks it is immensely important to give parents precise instructions and to start the exercises a few days before the surgical intervention in order to get parents and babies used to the procedure. It takes a lot of practice to perform sufficient wound management in such a small mouth, and many parents understandably have inhibitions about the fresh wound and a crying baby. If AWM is recommended, it should be performed four times a day (every 6 hours) for about 3 weeks. To do this, the person performing AMF positions himself or herself behind the head of the supine baby, places his or her clean index fingers to the right and left of the diamond-shaped wound, and lifts the tongue backward and upward. Finally, it should be mentioned that comprehensive care of the parents and the baby by a lactation consultant is useful, and sometimes the accompanying treatment by a myofunctional therapist and/or osteopath is necessary.

RESOURCES

There are some experts in the field of tongue-tie that provide a lot of knowledge on this subject. The book Tongue-Tied by Richard Baxter is the standard reference book on the issue. Furthermore, you can check the websites of Dr Bobby Ghaheri (www.drghaheri.com) and Dr Lawrence A. Kotlow (www.kiddsteeth.com), who provide a tremendous number of articles and data regarding that subject. Dr Soroush Zaghi even provides numerous educational YouTube videos of the procedure and also lectures that can be watched (www.zaghimd.com).

PARTICULAR CHALLENGES IN EVERYDAY PRACTICE

PMH AND MIH

Primary molar hypomineralization (PMH) and molar-incisor hypomineralization (MIH) pose a special challenge when treating children and adolescents. Reports of the prevalence of these defects vary widely across the world, ranging from 3% to 44%.[77]

Clinical features

Originally, the term *MIH* described a hypomineralization disorder confined to the permanent central incisors and the permanent first molars. However, this mineralization disorder has now been observed and described in relation to primary and other permanent teeth.

The mineralization disorder is based on a qualitative defect of the enamel where an increased amount of organic substance is present in otherwise inorganically mineralized

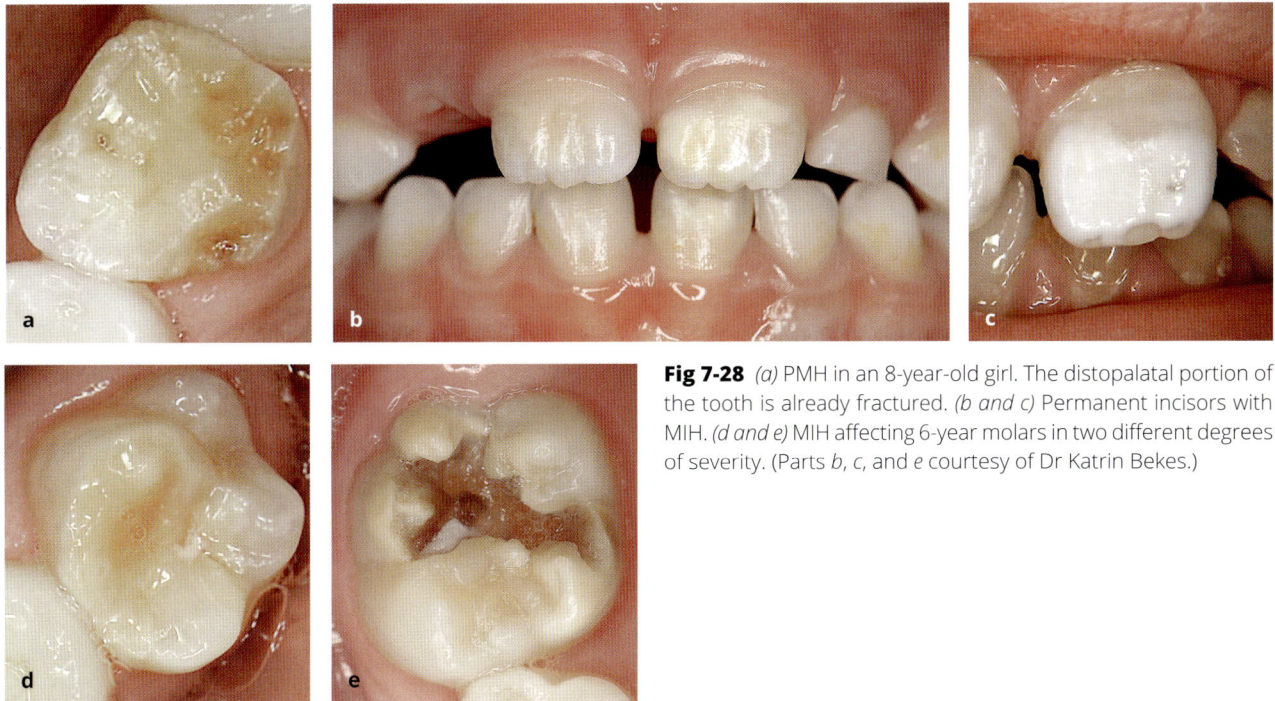

Fig 7-28 *(a)* PMH in an 8-year-old girl. The distopalatal portion of the tooth is already fractured. *(b and c)* Permanent incisors with MIH. *(d and e)* MIH affecting 6-year molars in two different degrees of severity. (Parts *b*, *c*, and *e* courtesy of Dr Katrin Bekes.)

enamel. Owing to this high protein content, which is up to 21 times higher than in regular enamel, affected areas of enamel are extremely porous and prone to fracture. Yellow, brown, or cream-colored opacities are the noticeable visual features. If MIH is less severe, it often only affects single permanent first molars and is evident as isolated, white to pale yellowish-looking enamel discolorations.

In severe cases of MIH, all the 6-year molars and the permanent incisors are involved. The enamel appears brownish, porous, and breaks off at the occluding cusp tips (Fig 7-28). This mineralization disorder is associated with considerable hypersensitivity of the teeth, which, even at lower degrees of severity, leads to reduced oral hygiene and diminished masticatory activity.[78]

Etiology

In terms of etiology, a multifactorial explanatory model is suggested, but there is no firm evidence. It is assumed that various factors have a negative impact on amelogenesis during natal development and up to 4 years of age. The following have been discussed as potential etiologic factors: premature births, dioxin-contaminated breast milk, complications in the last trimester of pregnancy, common diseases in infancy and preschool age (eg, high fever, respiratory diseases, middle ear infection, diarrhea), and increased exposure of the body to bisphenols.[79] The last of these factors is a growing focus of research.

Complications

One complication with PMH and MIH is that prevention in the classic sense is not possible. Only symptomatic and defect-focused therapy is available, which is made challenging by a variety of issues. The teeth are extremely sensitive to temperature and touch; simply drying the teeth during a routine dental checkup will cause pain in children affected by hypomineralization and, in some circumstances, may greatly reduce their willingness to undergo treatment and carry out thorough daily oral hygiene. At the same time, the relatively long eruption time of the 6-year molars makes it difficult to create a dry field during the treatment.

Furthermore, another challenge dentists face is inadequate pain elimination. Satisfactory freedom from pain during treatment often cannot be guaranteed by conventional anesthesia techniques, which obviously diminishes the child's compliance and hence the success of the treatment. Generally speaking, this phenomenon cannot be remedied by increasing the dose of local anesthetic.[79] This is mainly because the hypersensitivity exposes the pulp to chronic stress, which in turn means that inflammatory mediators, such as prostaglandins and bradykinins, will accumulate. This exposure alters the pH in the periapical tissue. Histamines and other inflammatory mediators produce a low pain threshold and make pain elimination more difficult.

In addition, the bond between classic composites and the hypomineralized areas of enamel is reduced and often leads to fractures in the marginal area of the filling or to the development of secondary caries. Very severe cases of MIH, in particular, are difficult to treat satisfactorily by conventional approaches in standard therapy (ie, without the possibility of sedation). To avoid failure, severe cases should be referred to specialists who have access to various sedation facilities.

Treatment

As a matter of principle, children affected by hypomineralization need to be involved in regular recall (every 3 months). The parents should be given dietary advice and especially tips on daily oral hygiene for their children (see chapter 3). A fluoride toothpaste containing at least 1,000 ppm fluoride should be used for the purposes of oral hygiene at home.[80] The author favors the use of a toothpaste with 1,500 ppm fluoride content. Regular use of Duraphat varnish (Colgate) and home application of CPP-ACP pastes has also proved effective in reducing hypersensitivity (for milder forms of MIH). Recent studies additionally suggest that arginine preparations are effective in decreasing tactile and thermal hypersensitivity.[81]

Treatment with SDF seems to be another option, although there are not yet any studies on its use for this indication. However, many dentists report very good personal experience with regard to reducing hypersensitivity. Nevertheless, the black discoloration has to be accepted as a negative side effect. All these measures are extremely important, especially in the initial posteruptive phase. If caries can be prevented at this stage, a great deal has been gained.

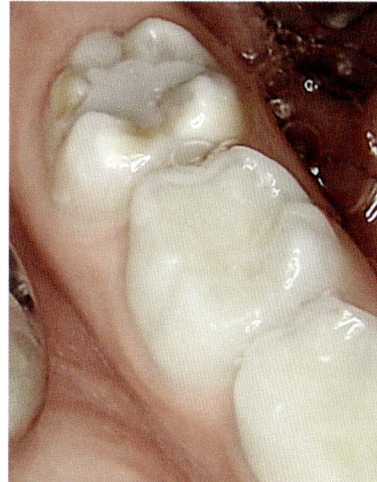

Fig 7-29 GIC sealing of permanent first molar, which exhibited severe hypersensitivity. The product used was Fuji Triage.

If children complain of pain as a result of hypomineralization, the teeth should be sealed with GIC or composite-reinforced GIC while still erupting (Fig 7-29). This reduces the pain sensitivity, which improves compliance and oral hygiene at home. Early carious damage can also be avoided.

While GIC sealing is a very effective transitional therapy, it is not a definitive solution. Fully erupted teeth with MIH and slight defects should be sealed at an early stage. Once again, treatment of hypersensitivities and prevention of caries are the priority. However, these measures do not minimize the risk of fracture.[78] If handled properly, composite restorations are also a reasonable treatment option (with an average survival rate of 5.2 years for teeth with MIH). Chipping fractures are relatively common because hypomineralized areas of enamel are sometimes difficult to locate and have a poorer adhesive bond. In studies, self-etch systems achieved better adhesion values than total-etch systems.[78] Another approach is to treat the affected teeth before filling placement with 5% NaOCl in order to eliminate organic constituents and improve the adhesion values. However, this is difficult to perform in practice.

Composite fillings must always be closely monitored in teeth with MIH in order to diagnose any fractures or marginal leakage at any early stage. Amalgam fillings are not suitable for restoration of teeth with MIH due to expansion upon hardening. For severely affected teeth that are very prone to fracture, a cemented molar band and early GIC sealing can provide additional stability.

A prefabricated SSC is another possible method of longer-term but still temporary restoration of teeth badly affected by MIH. By this method, the height of the bite can reliably be maintained. Unlike preparation in the primary dentition, preparation of the permanent molars should be as restrictive as possible or nonexistent, and, if possible, separation should not be performed. (Placement of orthodontic separating rubber bands can be helpful during this step.) Desensitization should be expected here because of the thick layer of cement placed under the SSC. For esthetic reasons, restoration with an SSC only offers a temporary solution and can later be replaced by a tooth-colored, laboratory-fabricated restoration. This is another reason to ensure the technique is as minimally invasive as possible. It is also possible to restore these teeth with prefabricated zirconia crowns. This will have by far a better esthetic result, but it requires a preparation and therefore results in the loss of tooth structure, which bears a disadvantage if the tooth has to be restored later.

Another therapeutic approach is to restore the teeth with laboratory-fabricated and fiberglass-reinforced composite restorations. These can also be banded, are esthetically attractive, and are repairable. It should be mentioned that computer-aided preparation of restorations is possible. However, the latter treatment options require a high level of compliance from the patient and parents. Extraction of severely affected teeth should be followed by orthodontic space closure.

Affected children who have had multiple visits to the dentist and a tooth already restored several times in childhood probably do not have a good long-term prognosis. The consequential costs in adulthood (eg, endodontics, implant dentistry) can quickly add up. In severe cases, extraction therapy is sometimes the better option if the primordia of the third molars can be safely identified by a panoramic radiograph. This obviously calls for an interdisciplinary therapeutic approach. The best extraction time is 10.5 years in the maxilla and between 8 and 11 years in the mandible.[78]

In the case of the primary teeth, it is primarily the severity of the lesion that matters. SSCs are excellently suited for severe cases and, as a result of the increased degree of attrition of the teeth, can often be used entirely without preparation or only after minimal approximal separation. Composite and compomer fillings can be used to treat less severe cases, while temporary GICs or composite-reinforced GICs are suitable for very young, rather uncooperative children or as a desensitizing measure.

> **TIP FOR PAIN ELIMINATION**
>
> The main problem with conservative treatment of teeth with MIH is that pain elimination is problematic. Among the available local anesthetics (lidocaine, mepivacaine, or articaine), none is superior to any other. Studies have shown that adequate pain elimination can be achieved with nerve block combined with intraligamentary anesthesia.[79] Furthermore, the administration of acetaminophen or ibuprofen prior to treatment has proved effective. Many authors favor administering ibuprofen 1 hour before the start of treatment in order to deepen the anesthetic effect, while other authors feel that an effect can
>
> ⟶

only be achieved if ibuprofen is started a few days beforehand, especially with respect to chronically inflamed pulp tissue.[79] Steffen and van Waes wrote that efficacious premedication requires very high doses of analgesic given only for a short period of time, that the analgesic should definitely have anti-inflammatory properties, and that four doses are needed before treatment.[82] These four doses should be given more than 24 hours before treatment, at 12 hours and 6 to 8 hours before treatment, and immediately prior to treatment. They recommend ibuprofen or acetaminophen as possible analgesics, and in very severe cases of hypersensitivity, both can be combined with a slight dose reduction. The author has had positive experiences with ibuprofen taken consistently every 6 hours, except at night, from 48 hours before the start of therapy (equivalent to three single doses in 24 hours according to the package leaflet, depending on the patient's weight). Admittedly, this is not a definitive treatment recommendation. Every patient has a unique response to these pain relievers, and the general medical history should be taken into account. In case of doubt, the relevant pediatrician should be consulted.

The MIH Treatment Need Index

The aim of the MIH treatment need index (MIH TNI), presented by Professor Katrin Bekes and colleagues, is to simplify standardized diagnostics and to establish the right therapeutic measures for dentists, depending on the severity of the lesion and the patient's risk of caries. Sometimes called the Würzburg MIH concept,[77,81] the MIH TNI can be used as a structured treatment recommendation, serves as a decision-making tool, and imparts confidence in dentists regarding treatment (Table 7-3). Based on the two clinically most significant symptoms, hypersensitivity and destruction, an initial classification can be made in order to determine MIH severity. The possible treatment can be deduced from this classification. The index applies equally to primary and permanent teeth. The treatment options deduced from the MIH TNI, depending on the individual caries risk, are summarized in Table 7-3.

TABLE 7-3 MIH TNI and treatment options

Index	Definition	Treatment options
0	No MIH, clinically healthy	
1	MIH without hypersensitivity, no substance defect	**Prophylaxis** • At home: Fluoride, tricalcium phosphate (TCP), CPP-ACP • In office: Varnish **Sealing** Fissure sealing (sealer or flowable) or GIC (low-viscosity)[a]
2	MIH without hypersensitivity, with substance defect	**Prophylaxis** • At home: Fluoride, TCP, CPP-ACP • In office: Varnish
2a	< $1/3$ defect extent	**Sealing** Fissure sealing (sealer or flowable) or GIC (low-viscosity) **Temporary restoration** GIC, GIC + orthoband, or SSC **Definitive restoration (after maturation)** Direct restoration (composite) or indirect restoration
2b	> $1/3$ < $2/3$ defect extent	**Temporary restoration** GIC, GIC + orthoband, or SSC **Definitive restoration (after maturation)** Direct restoration (composite) or indirect restoration
2c	> $2/3$ defect extent and/or defect close to pulp or extraction or atypical restoration	**Temporary restoration** GIC, GIC + orthoband, or SSC[b] **Definitive restoration (after maturation)** Direct restoration (composite) or indirect restoration **Other therapy** Extraction
3	MIH with hypersensitivity, without substance defect	**Prophylaxis** • At home: Fluoride, TCP, CPP-ACP • In office: Varnish **Sealing** Adhesive, fissure sealing (sealer or flowable), or GIC (low-viscosity) **Definitive restoration (after maturation)** Direct restoration (composite) or indirect restoration
4	MIH with hypersensitivity, with substance defect	**Prophylaxis** • At home: Fluoride, TCP, or CPP-ACP • In office: Varnish
4a	< $1/3$ extent	**Sealing** Adhesive, fissure sealing (sealer or flowable), or GIC (low-viscosity) **Temporary restoration** GIC, GIC + orthoband, or SSC **Definitive restoration (after maturation)** Direct restoration (composite) or indirect restoration
4b	> $1/3$ < $2/3$ extent	**Temporary restoration** GIC, GIC + orthoband, or SSC[c] **Definitive restoration (after maturation)** Direct restoration (composite) or indirect restoration
4c	> $2/3$ extent and/or defect close to pulp or extraction or atypical restoration	**Temporary restoration** GIC, GIC + orthoband, or SSC[b] **Definitive restoration (after maturation)** Direct restoration (composite) or indirect restoration **Other therapy** Extraction

[a]Only applies to patients with high caries risk; [b]does not apply to patients with high caries risk; [c]only applies to patients with low caries risk.

TRAUMA TO PRIMARY AND PERMANENT TEETH

Traumatic injuries, mainly to the permanent teeth, are among the most difficult cases in daily practice. Even though trauma is a relatively common occurrence, the routine experience in diagnosis and treatment needed to solve these complex cases really well is often still lacking, especially for the permanent teeth. This section is intended to give a brief overview and an insight into the strategies involved in treating trauma cases. After a few general facts, the management of primary tooth trauma is discussed, followed by the permanent teeth in the same sequence.

In terms of prophylaxis, apart from the fabrication of protective splints for children involved in high-risk sports, myofunctional and orthodontic treatment of malpositioned teeth is important. Children with protrusion of the maxillary anterior teeth and incompetent lip closure have an increased risk of anterior dental trauma.[83]

A systematic approach is important when treating trauma-damaged teeth, regardless of whether they are primary or permanent teeth.[84] Preprinted forms for recording dental trauma are helpful in documenting what is also forensically significant, especially for permanent teeth (www.aapd.org/globalassets/media/policies_guidelines/r_acutetrauma. pdf). There is a really recommendable app called AcciDent that guides the practitioner through the treatment step by step.[85] A structured guide gives the dentist confidence to cope with unfamiliar situations and ensures that the parents are asked for all the relevant information. This app can be downloaded at www.dget.de/fuer-zahnaerzte/traumaapp and the language changed to English.

While gathering patient history, dentists should inquire about a few key points about the circumstances of the accident in order to establish the time sequence between the traumatic event and attendance at the dental practice. Questions should be asked about the circumstances of the accident in order to obtain information about possible contamination of the wound. It is important to check for evidence of a head injury (ie, loss of consciousness, headache, nausea, vomiting, and amnesia), and the parents must be made aware of the possibility.[84] In the case of trauma-related injuries, the patient history should include tetanus vaccination status. If a third party is responsible for the trauma (eg, another driver in a car accident or the school where the trauma took place), outside insurance claims may be filed to cover the costs, so it is always wise to know exactly where and when the accident occurred.

After a thorough history has been documented, dentists should perform an extraoral and intraoral examination. The documentation can be complemented with photographs, if that is a possibility. The adjacent soft and hard tissues should be examined in the extraoral examination. If tooth or bone fragments cannot be found, but adjacent soft tissues are injured and swollen, it may be that these fragments have become displaced into the soft tissues. This has to be verified by radiographs. Furthermore, function should be checked, which means excluding a malocclusion due to displaced teeth and checking the mobility of the mouth and jaws. In the case of chin injuries, a panoramic radiograph should be taken to exclude a condylar neck fracture.

The intraoral examination should include pulp testing, percussion tests, palpation of adjacent tissue, and clinical examination of the teeth, periodontium, and bone. In terms of radiographic examinations, dental radiographs, occlusal films, or a panoramic radiograph may be considered. Occlusal views are recommended mainly to exclude root fractures, while a panoramic radiograph is primarily indicated for diagnostic assessment of the temporomandibular joints. The stage of root growth, dislocation of teeth or fragments, or the path of the periodontal space can be assessed on intraoral radiographs. Root fractures appear as an elliptic radiolucent double contour on a standard dental radiograph.

If a child repeatedly attends with dental injuries, practitioners should watch for signs of domestic violence. A dentist should always be skeptical if:

• A lengthy period of time elapses between the accident and attendance at the dental practice.
• The child has several bruises that differ in color and hence in age.
• The account of the circumstances of the accident does not match the clinical findings.
• Parents and child give very different details of what happened.

The titanium trauma splint (TTS) is really useful when treating dental traumas. It provides strength and can be bent manually and adapted to the dental arch but equally allows physiologic mobility.[86] The slender splint is fixed using self-etch adhesives and composite, which make it easy to remove. It is advisable not to use a tooth-colored composite but rather a composite like Tetric Flow Bleach (Ivoclar Vivadent), as this makes removal much easier. Furthermore, every dental practice should have access to a tooth rescue box so that dehydrated or nonphysiologically stored teeth or tooth fragments can be deposited and rehydrated before further treatment. Some other useful things for successful management of a dental trauma in the dental practice include MTA (preferably nonstaining and white[87]), Ledermix (Sigma), and Odontopaste (ADM).

BASIC PROCEDURE FOR ANY DENTAL TRAUMA
1. Keep calm and reassure the parents and child.
2. Take a history of the circumstances of the accident.
3. Inspect and palpate the teeth concerned to check the degree of looseness and integrity.
4. If possible and necessary, perform radiographic examination.
5. Depending on the findings, carry out necessary treatments.

ADVICE TO PARENTS WHO CALL AFTER A DENTAL TRAUMA
• Stay calm
• Stop the bleeding by applying pressure with a compress or a clean handkerchief
• Cool the injury

$\longrightarrow$

- Leave loose and/or dislodged teeth in place
- Look for knocked-out teeth, pick up by the crown of the tooth and not the root, and do not clean but keep moist (if there is no tooth rescue box available, then it can be stored in milk)
- Come into the office at once

Management of primary tooth trauma

With a prevalence of approximately 45%, primary tooth traumas are very common. Injuries to the primary anterior teeth are not a rarity, especially at the toddler stage. Unfortunately, it is often the case that a trauma may well be the first time parents have a reason for taking their child to a dentist. This makes the already difficult treatment of small patients even more problematic. The priorities when treating primary tooth trauma are to eliminate pain and prevent damage to the tooth germ. The treatment should be as straightforward and practical as possible. While complex tooth-preserving treatments are presented below, in the author's opinion these have little practical relevance in the primary dentition. The rule "extract or do nothing" frequently applies. Kirschner et al write: "Indicated surgical treatments are always performed under local anesthesia. Treatments under endotracheal anesthesia following dental trauma in the primary dentition are basically inappropriate."[86] This obviously does not apply to soft tissue injuries and/ or fractures requiring treatment.

Unfortunately, it is often the case that a trauma may well be the first time parents have a reason for taking their child to a dentist.

Crown fractures

Enamel fractures require no treatment or, with satisfactory cooperation, only smoothing of sharp edges.

Uncomplicated coronal fractures, meaning without pulp exposure, should, if possible, be covered with composites or compomers in order to seal the dentin.

Teeth with *complicated coronal fractures* and therefore showing pulp exposure, depending on the age and compliance of the patient, are either treated endodontically (pulpotomy) or extracted if cooperation is poor and/or the child is older than 4 years. If cooperation is entirely inadequate and the tooth is still firmly fixed, brief sedation with a specialist may be considered. For loose primary anterior teeth, the application of a surface anesthetic, distraction of the child, and the speed of an experienced practitioner in removing the tooth might be sufficient in some cases.

The rule "extract or do nothing" frequently applies.

Crown-root fractures

The presence of vertical crown-root fractures always requires extraction of the primary tooth, except in the case of slightly supragingival fractures without pulp involvement.

Root fractures

There are various recommendations in the literature regarding horizontal root fractures. If the coronal fragment is not displaced and not too badly loosened, it can merely be

Fig 7-30 Deep-lying transverse root fracture of a primary anterior tooth; the tooth showed only a looseness grade of 1, and there was no communication with the oral cavity. In this case, everything was left alone and regularly checked.

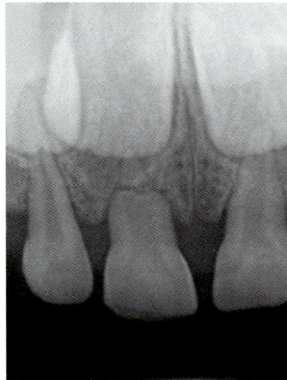

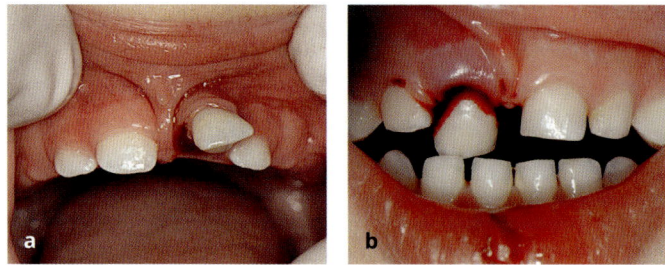

Fig 7-31 Dislocated primary teeth where extraction is indicated. *(a)* Severely dislocated maxillary primary left central incisor. *(b)* Dislocated maxillary primary right central incisor that is now an occlusal obstacle. (Courtesy of Dr Gabriele Viergutz.)

monitored (Fig 7-30). If the coronal fragment is dislodged or severely loosened, this part of the tooth must be removed. If there is no connection between the root fragment and the oral cavity (ie, the transverse fracture lies in the apical third), the apical fragment can be left in place. This approach is debated in the literature.[85,86] Because extraction of an apical root fragment without damaging the tooth germ is only possible with very good compliance, the author would advise leaving the apical part of the root if there is no risk of infection.

Dislocation injuries

In dislocation injuries, tooth preservation only makes sense if an injury to the tooth germ can be excluded and the child is sufficiently cooperative for necessary treatments. The asymmetric position of adjacent tooth germs on the radiograph is evidence of tooth germ damage. In this case, the primary teeth concerned should be extracted.

Bidigital compression of the extraction wounds should be omitted after extraction of traumatized primary teeth in order to prevent blood being pressed into a potentially injured dental follicle.[86]

Concussion and/or loosening. A checkup is all that is required in this instance (see "Education, prescribing, and recall").

Lateral dislocation of primary teeth. Primary teeth that are only slightly dislocated and show no malocclusion in habitual intercuspation can simply be left in place. Significantly dislocated primary teeth that are still relatively stable and where damage to the tooth germ can be excluded can be repositioned under local anesthesia if compliance is very good; if necessary, they can be splinted on the day of the accident. That being said, the author refrains from splinting primary teeth. If compliance is poor, extraction tends to be indicated, for which premedication might be necessary if there is a lack of compliance. Figure 7-31 shows dislocated primary teeth where extraction is indicated.

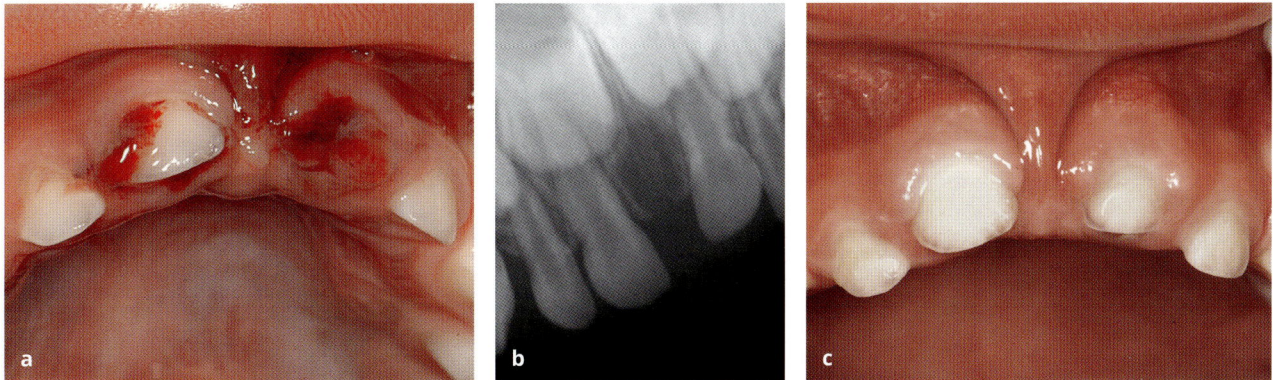

Fig 7-32 *(a)* It cannot be ascertained simply from this finding whether the primary left central incisor is avulsed or completely intruded. *(b)* The radiograph provides clarity: It is a matter of complete intrusion. *(c)* Reeruption of the primary left central incisor visible after 1 week. (Courtesy of Dr Gabriele Viergutz.)

CAUTION WITH DISLOCATIONS

If the primary tooth crown has been displaced labially and consequently the primary tooth root is displaced palatally, there is a risk of damage to the tooth germ. In this case the dislocated primary tooth must be extracted to avoid infection of the follicle.[86] Radiographically, a primary tooth root displaced palatally in the direction of the tooth germ appears lengthened on radiographs. If the root of the injured primary tooth is shortened on radiographs, it may be assumed that the primary tooth root has been dislocated labially, and hence it has not injured the tooth germ. In this case (see Fig 7-31), the primary tooth crown was consequently displaced lingually.

Intrusion injuries. If a tooth germ injury can be excluded by radiography, it is possible to wait for secondary eruption in the case of primary tooth intrusion (see Fig 7-32c). Extraction is indicated if the primary tooth shows no tendency to reerupt after 4 weeks and if tooth germ damage is suspected. This may be radiographically evident as an asymmetric position of the tooth germs, for instance. Primary teeth can certainly intrude completely. In cases where parents have not found the tooth, it is hence absolutely necessary to take a radiograph to distinguish between complete intrusion and avulsion (Fig 7-32).

Extrusion injuries. If extrusion of a primary tooth is minimal, a wait-and-see approach can be adopted. In the case of severe loosening, the primary tooth should be extracted. Careful repositioning and splinting on the day of the accident are possible if compliance is excellent. Kirschner et al describe a replantation technique associated with the endodontic treatment of severely extruded or avulsed primary teeth.[86] However, in the author's opinion it is highly doubtful whether the risk-benefit relationship of this approach is balanced for primary anterior teeth, which enter the physiologic resorption phase after only 4 years and where unsatisfactory patient compliance must be assumed beforehand.

Avulsion injuries. In the case of completely avulsed primary teeth, the author would not perform replantation for the above reasons. Kirschner et al do state that avulsed primary teeth stored in cell-physiologic conditions can be replanted, provided root growth is not yet completed. If the latter is true, the avulsed primary tooth can be endodontically treated extraorally from the apical direction (root canal filling with calcium hydroxide) and subsequently replanted and splinted.[86] However, the author considers this approach irrelevant for practical purposes.

> **CAUTION ABOUT SUSPECTED AVULSION**
> If a small patient with a trauma-related gap between the teeth attends the practice and the tooth concerned cannot be found, complete intrusion of the tooth must be excluded radiographically before avulsion is confirmed.

Alveolar process fractures

Nearly every tooth trauma goes hand in hand with injuries to the socket. Simple contusions sustained during the course of injuries treated as described above do not require separate treatment. If individual small bone fragments are mobile but joined to the periosteum, they do not necessarily have to be removed. Extensive injuries to the alveolar bone must be treated in a specialist clinic or by a surgically experienced colleague.

Soft tissue injuries in infants/children

Bite injuries and tearing of the labial frenum are very often seen in cases of trauma. These injuries are usually uncomplicated and most do not require separate treatment. Small wounds, the margins of which can be classified as smooth and sound, can be repaired with atraumatic sutures (5/0 or 6/0). Contaminated wounds are rinsed with physiologic saline. Injuries to the vermilion of the lip should always be treated by a surgical specialist because of the special esthetic challenge involved.

> **OVERVIEW OF TRAUMA TO PRIMARY TEETH**
> The treatment of primary tooth trauma varies depending on the nature of the injury and patient compliance. Elimination of pain, prevention of damage to tooth germs, and care of any wounds are the crucial elements. The treatment should be appropriate, and the risk should not outweigh the benefit. This is why the rule of "extract or do nothing" often applies in cases of primary tooth trauma.[84] In the majority of cases, children attend the practice with mild concussion or dislocation and soft tissue injuries (eg, the torn labial frenum is a classic injury). Commonly, nothing at all needs to be done in these cases. When damage is severe, extraction is often the method of choice. Splinting is possible in principle and has been described in the relevant sections, but it tends not to be the rule in daily practice. Box 7-1 provides the treatment options for managing trauma to primary teeth.

BOX 7-1 Treatment options for primary tooth trauma

ALWAYS take an initial radiograph and establish short recall intervals!

Uncomplicated crown fracture
- In enamel: Possible smoothing, fluoridation
- In dentin: Adhesive filling

Complicated crown fracture
- With very good cooperation and under 4 years: Pulpotomy with MTA or calcium hydroxide
- With poor cooperation or over 4 years: Extraction

Crown-root fracture
- Extraction

Root fracture
- If the coronal fragment is not too loose and there is no communication between the fracture gap and the oral cavity: Leave in place and observe
- If the coronal fragment is severely loosened: Removal of fragment (the root apex can be left if it does not communicate directly with the oral cavity; ie, the transverse fracture lies in the apical third)

Concussion/looseness
- Monitoring

Lateral dislocation
- For dislocation of the crown in the labial direction: Extraction (because it will displace the root palatally and damage the tooth germ)
- For dislocation of the crown in the palatal direction with good cooperation: Cautious repositioning under local anesthesia
- For very minimal dislocation and normal occlusion: Leave in place and observe
- With minimal cooperation and severe dislocation and/or risk of tooth germ damage: Extraction (ALWAYS)

Intrusion
- If tooth germ damage is suspected: Extraction
- If tooth germ damage can be excluded: Await spontaneous reeruption
- If no tendency for reeruption after 4 weeks: Extraction

Extrusion
- Minimal extrusion: Wait
- Severe extrusion: Extraction

Avulsion
- Wound care
- Exclude possible complete intrusion by radiograph
- **It is not recommended to replant avulsed primary teeth**

RESOURCE ON MANAGING TRAUMA

The American Academy of Pediatric Dentistry (AAPD) has an excellent resource on managing trauma in primary teeth. Detailed illustrations of the possible injuries and their relevant treatment and recall options are presented: https://www.aapd.org/media/Policies_Guidelines/E_Injuries.pdf.

Fig 7-33 *(a)* Sustained discoloration of the maxillary primary right central incisor after preceding trauma. *(b)* Almost complete obliteration of the pulp cavity can clearly be seen. There are no signs of inflammation, so natural exfoliation can calmly be awaited. (Courtesy of Dr Juliane von Hoyningen-Huene.)

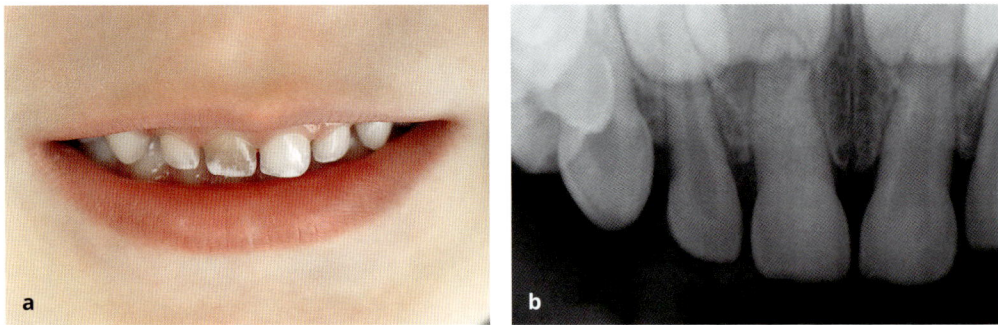

Education, prescribing, and recall

It is important to explain possible consequences to parents in the course of a primary tooth trauma. The following are relatively common:

- Discolorations (may have different causes; the discoloration is often reversible if due to bleeding, but not in the case of obliteration or pulp necrosis); prevalence approximately 50% (Fig 7-33)
- Pulp necrosis; prevalence approximately 25%
- Pulp obliteration; prevalence approximately 30%

If apical periodontitis and/or fistulae develop, the primary tooth must be extracted in order to avoid damage to the tooth germ. This can manifest itself in permanent teeth as the following:

- Opacities of the dental enamel
- Eruptive disorders
- Deformation of the dental crown
- Dilacerations
- Hypoplasias

The risk of tooth germ damage declines with age and is highest with intrusion injuries.[83] Figure 7-34 shows enamel hypoplasia, an amelogenesis disorder, and a structural anomaly following primary tooth trauma.

Depending on the degree of injury, soft food should be prescribed after a dental trauma. Intuitively, children often bite off food sideways and avoid hard foods. The parents must be required to ensure thorough oral hygiene. In the case of splinting or more severe injuries, an alcohol-free CHX mouthwash may additionally be prescribed

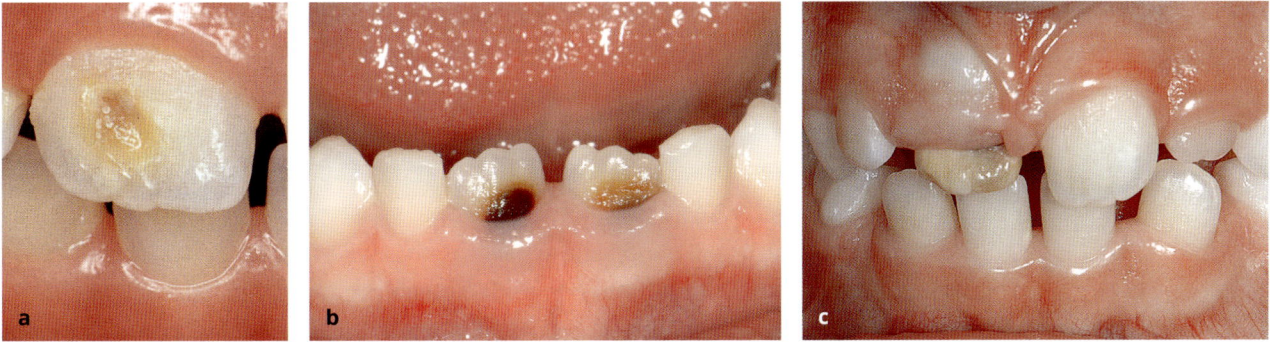

Fig 7-34 *(a)* Enamel hypoplasia. *(b)* Amelogenesis disorder. *(c)* Structural anomaly. (Courtesy of Dr Gabriele Viergutz.)

for a week. Following intrusion injuries, children should not be offered a pacifier until spontaneous reeruption happens.

The following recall intervals are recommended: reattendance after 1, 2, 4, and 6 weeks; after 3 and 6 months; and then annually until natural exfoliation occurs. The parents must be made aware of the possibility of fistula formation and told that it is a reason for immediate reattendance and extraction of the affected tooth.

Management of permanent tooth trauma

The priorities when treating dental trauma involving permanent teeth are the preservation of vital pulp, completion of root growth, healing of the periodontium, preservation/restoration of the esthetics, and obviously tooth preservation. Crucial factors regarding tooth preservation are, above all, the time between the accident and first attendance at the dentist office, the maturity of the root, the degree of injury, and, in the case of avulsions, storage of the tooth until the patient attends the practice.

> **NOTES**
> - A negative pulp test on the actual day of the accident does not necessarily mean necrosis of the pulp if the injury is not very dramatic. It may also involve a reversible loss of sensitivity, which is caused by edema or hematoma, for example.
> - Discoloration immediately after trauma tends to suggest a reversible color change due to bleeding. If a discoloration does not appear until a few weeks or months later, it must be assumed that pulp necrosis has occurred. For this reason, regular clinical and radiographic follow-up with short recall intervals is essential (see "Education, prescribing, and recall" on page 159).

When splinting is mentioned in the following section, it refers to flexible fixation of the affected tooth with adhesive, flowable composite (not tooth-colored) and TTS, together with an adjacent unaffected tooth. This type of flexible splinting is recommended for all injuries, except an alveolar process fracture (in these cases, rigid splinting is performed involving two adjacent unaffected teeth). The duration of splinting differs depending on the nature of the injury (see below in the individual subsections).

For avulsions, intrusions, and severe dislocations, systemic administration of doxycycline for 7 days is additionally recommended. More details of dosage and age specifications are given in the section "Antibiotic Use in Children."

Generally speaking, a dental radiograph must always be taken, even if no dislocation injury is apparent. This is the only way to exclude root fractures or similar problems.

Crown fractures

Enamel fractures require no treatment or, at most, smoothing of sharp edges. Fluoridation and pulp testing should be carried out.

Uncomplicated crown fractures without pulp exposure require a small filling. For larger hard tissue losses, it may be advisable to reattach the existing fragment. For this purpose, the fragment should not have been kept in dry conditions in the interim. If it has, the piece of tooth must be rehydrated beforehand (eg, placed in physiologic saline for several hours or, better, in a tooth rescue box and reattached the following day). For recementation, the tooth and fragment should be treated by acid etching and bonding; the bonding agent should not be light cured in order to guarantee a better fit between tooth and fragment. Flowable composites are suitable as composite. In any event, the dentin wound should be covered even if the definitive restoration cannot take place until the next day. According to Weiger et al, easily removable materials such as light-cured calcium hydroxide cement are particularly suitable.[85] Root fractures should be radiographically excluded.

Teeth with *complicated crown fractures*—ie, with pulp exposure—must be treated as quickly as possible. If patients attend the dentist's immediately after the accident, small exposed areas can be treated by direct capping (up to 2 hours post-trauma). This can be done either with MTA or a calcium hydroxide preparation. Only a white, nonstaining MTA should be used for anterior teeth because otherwise a gray discoloration of the teeth will appear after just a few weeks. If the pulp is extensively or already exposed for more than 2 hours but less than 2 days, a partial pulpotomy should be performed (including teeth whose root growth is already completed). Partial pulpotomy means that the coronal pulp is amputated around 2 to 3 mm deep. This should be done under saline cooling with a diamond at high speed. Bleeding from the pulp wound should stop after a maximum of 5 minutes without hemostatic agents. The wound is also covered with a white MTA or calcium hydroxide preparation, then layered with a light-cured calcium hydroxide cement and finally restored with an adhesive filling or adhesive reattachment of the fragment.

If the wound is open for longer than 48 hours, a deeper pulpotomy may be attempted (Fig 7-35). Root canal treatment (RCT) is only rarely necessary, but it becomes more likely if there is an additional, more severe dislocation.

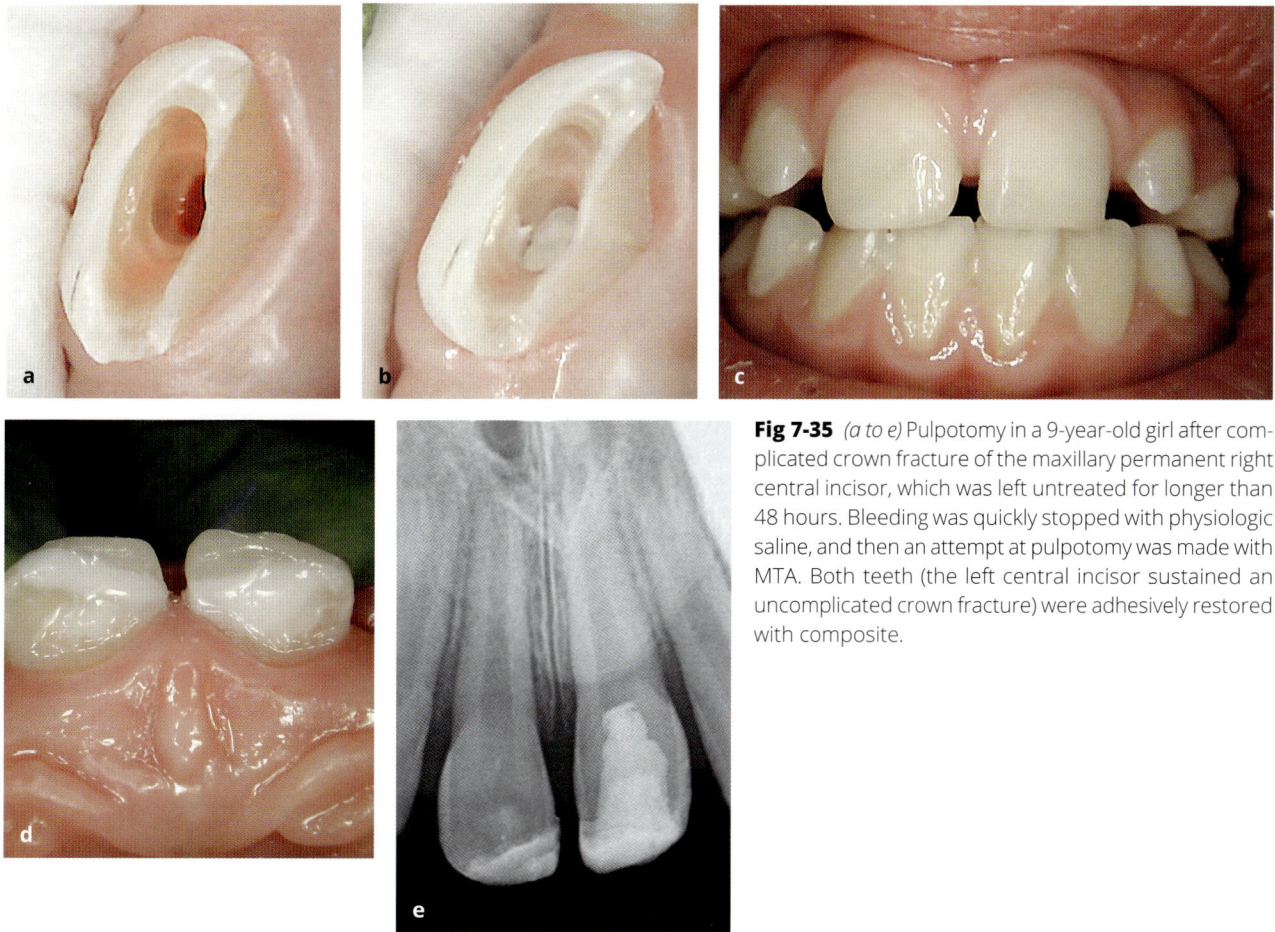

Fig 7-35 *(a to e)* Pulpotomy in a 9-year-old girl after complicated crown fracture of the maxillary permanent right central incisor, which was left untreated for longer than 48 hours. Bleeding was quickly stopped with physiologic saline, and then an attempt at pulpotomy was made with MTA. Both teeth (the left central incisor sustained an uncomplicated crown fracture) were adhesively restored with composite.

Crown-root fractures

Crown-root fractures, depending on the depth of defect, are very challenging and difficult to treat. Long-term restoration is difficult, especially if there are deeply subgingival fracture lines. Preserving the tooth until implant placement becomes possible can often be seen as a success in young patients.[85]

Additional root fractures should first be radiographically excluded. Fragments, often still with slight gingival attachment, must be removed. Depending on whether the pulp is affected, treatment is the same as for an (un)complicated crown fracture, except that subgingival defect borders must be made accessible (gingivectomy, osteotomy, and if deeper than 4 mm subgingivally by surgical or orthodontic extrusion as well). If the tooth is fractured too deeply, extraction is the only possibility. Furthermore Weiger et al refer to another treatment option where only the supragingival surfaces undergo restoration and subgingival defects are left alone.[85]

Root fractures

Root fractures are difficult to diagnose radiographically. In favorable circumstances, they present as an elliptical radiolucency that appears as a double contour due to projection of the oblique fracture gap.

The coronal tooth fragment may be loosened and displaced. If the fracture is so deep that communication of the fracture gap with the oral cavity can be excluded, the coronal fragment should be repositioned and splinted with TTS and composite for 4 weeks. If the coronal fragment is more severely loosened, the splinting time may be extended to as much as 12 weeks.[85]

Even if there is no reaction to pulp testing, it is possible to wait and see. Pulp regeneration takes place in most cases (the chance does decrease with the increasing degree of dislocation). Obliteration of the coronal fragment should be classified as a form of regeneration. Provided there is no evidence of pulp necrosis or signs of resorption, endodontic treatment does not have to be carried out. If pain, sensitivity to percussion, loosening of the coronal fragment, and anomalies on the radiograph are observed, RCT of the coronal fragment is recommended.

Dislocation injuries

Concussion and/or loosening. The teeth are usually sensitive to touch and percussion and can be splinted for 2 weeks for pain reduction. If pulp testing is negative, a wait-and-see approach is recommended. Endodontic treatment is only indicated if pulp necrosis or resorption later develop.

Lateral dislocation. A widened periodontal ligament space is evident on radiographs. The initial pulp testing is often negative, and sulcular bleeding is observed.

According to Weiger et al, the most common type of dislocation of anterior teeth is in the lingual direction.[85] The tooth should be carefully repositioned under local anesthesia. It should then be splinted for 2 to 4 weeks. The more severe the dislocation was, the more likely RCT becomes. If root growth is completed and the dislocation is more than 1 mm, pulp regeneration is improbable. Systemic doxycycline administration for 7 days is additionally recommended for severe dislocation injuries of more than 5-mm displacement.

CAUTION ABOUT LATERAL DISLOCATION
The thin, vestibular bone lamella is often fractured by labial dislocation of the root if the crown is dislocated lingually. Wedging of the root apex at the fracture line of the vestibular bone can occur in the process. To release the tooth from this wedging, exert gentle finger pressure on the vestibular bone lamella during repositioning, directed occlusally (Fig 7-36).

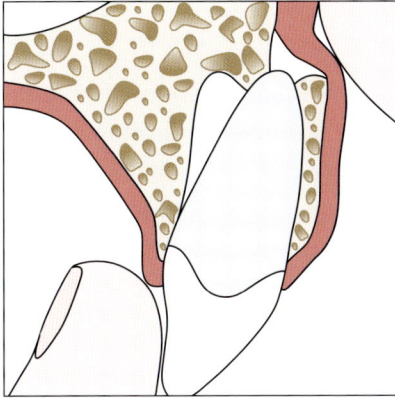

Fig 7-36 Vestibular wedging of the root apex, which is released by slight finger pressure from vestibular to occlusal.

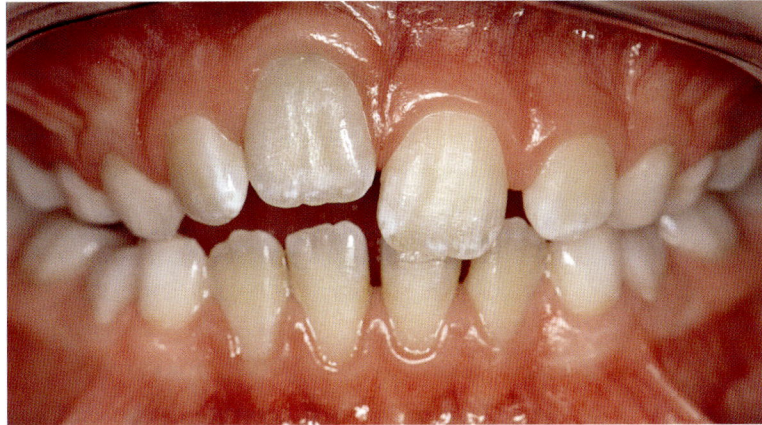

Fig 7-37 Ankylosis and infraposition of the maxillary permanent right central incisor. (Courtesy of Dr Gabriele Viergutz.)

Intrusion injuries. Intrusion injuries have a very poor prognosis because the periodontium and the alveolar bone are severely injured due to compression of the endodontium. Initial pulp testing is often negative, and radiographs frequently show an interrupted periodontal space apically when the affected tooth is in an infraposition.

For intrusion injuries, repositioning should be performed with forceps under local anesthesia. If spontaneous reeruption is awaited, ankylosis of the intruded tooth may occur, with considerable esthetic impairment. This can cause major problems, especially in terms of soft tissue management during later extraction and implant placement (Fig 7-37). This is why immediate repositioning should be performed, particularly when teeth have mature roots. If the patient does not attend until a few days later, orthodontic extrusion may be considered.

After repositioning, the tooth is splinted for 2 to 4 weeks, RCT is initiated with Ledermix dressing for 1 to 2 weeks, and doxycycline is prescribed for 7 days. Intrusions nearly always lead to resorption, which is why speedy initiation of endodontic treatment is advisable. The prognosis is rather better for teeth with immature roots.

Extrusion injuries. Clinically, an elongated tooth is evident, which might even pose an obstacle to occlusion. Pulp testing is often negative, while radiographs show a widened periodontal ligament space. In a case of extrusion, the tooth should be carefully repositioned with slow finger pressure. This is followed by splinting for 2 weeks. If extrusion is minimal and/or the apex is open, RCT does not have to be carried out immediately. An initially negative pulp test is not unusual and can be monitored. If root growth is completed, endodontic therapy should take place early for extrusion, provided the degree of extrusion is not slight.

Avulsion injuries. Avulsion injuries are a dental emergency and concern roughly 0.5% to 3% of all injuries to the permanent teeth.[83] A tooth rescue box is the best place to store knocked-out teeth. Tooth rescue boxes can be found in most schools and nurseries. Dental practices should always have a tooth rescue box because storing a tooth in this solution prior to replantation is part of antiresorptive regenerative therapy and promotes periodontal healing. If available, NoResorb (Medcem) should be added to the fluid in the tooth rescue box.[85] This is a mixture of tetracycline and dexamethasone, filled into capsules. The aim is to ensure survival of the cells on the root surface and prevent resorption and ankylosis. Generally speaking, doxycycline should be administered systemically for 7 days in the case of avulsions. Flexible splinting lasts for 2 weeks. If teeth have been stored in dry conditions for more than 1 hour, the splinting time should be extended up to 4 weeks.

The best treatment for avulsion is definitely immediate replantation at the site of the accident, possibly after any contamination has been cleaned off under cold, running water. If a patient then attends the practice later, the tooth should be left in place, radiographed, and splinted for 2 weeks. If teeth have a wide-open apex, endodontic treatment does not have to be performed immediately because revascularization might occur. Teeth with mature roots should undergo endodontic treatment without delay (ie, after splint placement). Trephination and Ledermix dressing for 1 to 2 weeks takes place first, followed by another dressing with calcium hydroxide. Root filling should be performed after 4 to 8 weeks.

Odontopaste can also be used as an initial dressing to prevent discolorations at a later stage. Among its ingredients, Odontopaste contains clindamycin and the anti-inflammatory active substance triamcinolone acetonide, and it is white in color. By contrast, Ledermix is based on demeclocycline (a tetracycline) and is grayish-green in color.

Teeth that are not immediately replanted have a worse prognosis, which is largely dependent on the storage medium. In these cases, as soon as the patient arrives the tooth should be placed in a tooth rescue box during the preparation time, ideally with added NoResorb. A contaminated root surface must be cleaned carefully with saline before replantation. The tooth should only be gripped by the crown. Any blood clot in the socket must be removed before replantation. The socket can equally be irrigated with saline. Replantation should be performed slowly with as little pressure as possible. For teeth with mature roots, immediate endodontic therapy after splinting is performed as described above.

When teeth have a wide-open apex, the start of endodontic treatment is dependent on the storage medium and the time elapsed. If the tooth has been stored in moist conditions (eg, milk, nutrient medium) or no more than 1 hour in dry storage has yet elapsed, it is possible to wait and see. In the case of dry storage and a longer time window (more than 1 hour), it may be assumed that the cells of the periodontal ligament are destroyed, even when teeth have immature roots. In this case, it is advisable to initiate endodontic treatment immediately. Because root treatment and filling of teeth with a wide-open apex pose a challenge, interdisciplinary cooperation with an endodontic specialist is advisable. The purpose is apexification, which means the formation of a barrier of hard substance at the apex. As a very long-term calcium hydroxide dressing over several months increases the fracture risk, apical closure with MTA followed by root filling with gutta-percha and a sealer is preferred. During treatment, rinsing should be done with sodium hypochlorite with ultrasound activation, if possible.

Paradigm shift in the treatment of immature, nonvital teeth
The subject of revascularization should briefly be addressed. The great problem posed by teeth with immature roots and a large lumen is the thin walls of the root canals with inadequate dentin thickness. Regardless of whether apexification is attempted with calcium hydroxide or apical MTA plug and subsequent root canal filling, the dentin walls remain thin and fragile. In the technique of revascularization, nonvital immature teeth are regenerated: After disinfection of the canal and placement of an antibiotic paste, stem cells from the apical region are introduced into the canal by means of bleeding provoked by the dental practitioner. This technique can also be applied for gangrenous, fistulating teeth or teeth with apical radiolucencies.[88] Unlike a definitive root filling with apical MTA plug and gutta-percha, the advantage of this method of regenerative endodontics is that apical root growth is brought to a conclusion, and, secondly, an increase in dentin wall thickness and hence stabilization are achieved. Therefore, revascularization is intended to revitalize a nonvital tooth and, in the best case, leads to a vital tooth whose root growth is completed.[89] This treatment approach, however, must be undertaken by a colleague specializing in endodontics under surgical microscope.

Alveolar process fractures and soft tissue injuries
The treatment for these injuries is the same as for primary teeth (see previous section).

OVERVIEW OF TRAUMA TO PERMANENT TEETH
Injuries to permanent teeth are unquestionably dental emergencies and must be treated without delay. They always pose a special challenge to the practice team. In this regard, important factors are a structured procedure, thorough history-taking and diagnostic assessment, possibly interdisciplinary cooperation with endodontists and/or surgeons, and, last but not least, a detailed explanation to the parents of any delayed effects and short recall intervals. Box 7-2 provides the treatment options for managing trauma to permanent teeth.

Education, prescribing, and recall
Regular follow-up after dental trauma is extremely important and includes taking dental radiographs as well as pulp and percussion testing. The recommended follow-up intervals are after 1, 3, 6, and 12 months. After that, there should be annual checkups for at least 5 years. In the case of very severe trauma, with likely resorption processes (ie, intrusions, avulsions, or severe lateral dislocations), checking radiographs at shorter intervals might be indicated.

BOX 7-2 Treatment options for permanent tooth trauma

ALWAYS take an initial radiograph and establish short recall intervals with pulp testing and radiographs!

Uncomplicated crown fracture
- In enamel: Possible smoothing, fluoridation
- In dentin: Adhesive filling or reattachment of fragment

Complicated crown fracture
- Objective: Preserve vitality
- Shortly after trauma (up to 2 hours) or small exposure: Direct capping with MTA or calcium hydroxide
- Large pulp exposure or longer than 2 hours after trauma: Partial pulpotomy
- Trauma more than 48 hours ago: Attempt deep pulpotomy, but RCT is more likely

Crown-root fracture
- Objective: Tooth preservation
- Removal of loose fragments
- In case of pulp exposure: See "Complicated crown fracture"
- Expose subgingival defect borders
- If absolutely no restoration possible: Extraction

Root fracture
- Objective: Preserve vitality and tooth
- If the coronal fragment communicates with the oral cavity, its preservation is not possible (possible extraction of root)
- If the coronal fragment has no connection with the oral cavity: Repositioning and TTS splinting for 4 to 12 weeks (depending on the degree of looseness)
- If signs of pulp necrosis or resorption: Coronal fragment must undergo RCT
- Obliteration of the coronal fragment should be viewed as regeneration

Concussion/looseness
- Objective: Preserve vitality
- Splinting with TTS for pain reduction for 2 weeks

Lateral dislocation
- Objective: Tooth preservation
- Repositioning
- Splinting with TTS for pain reduction for 2 to 4 weeks
- If dislocation is over 1 mm and root growth is completed: RCT becomes more likely
- If discoloration is over 2 mm: Doxycycline administration for 7 days in addition to RCT

Intrusion
- Objective: Tooth preservation
- Repositioning
- Splinting with TTS for pain reduction for 2 to 4 weeks
- RCT with initial Ledermix dressing for 1 to 2 weeks
- Doxycycline administration for 7 days

Extrusion
- Objective: Preserve vitality and tooth
- Repositioning
- Splinting with TTS for 2 weeks
- Minimal extrusion and incomplete root growth: Wait
- Pronounced extrusion and completed root growth: Initiate RCT early

Avulsion
- Objective: Tooth preservation
- Place tooth in the rescue box for 30 minutes, if possible with NoResorb
- Replantation
- Splinting with TTS for pain reduction for 2 to 4 weeks
- Teeth with immature roots: Wait, but monitor closely!
- Teeth with mature roots: Immediate RCT with initial Ledermix dressing for 1 to 2 weeks
- Doxycycline administration for 7 days

The following are delayed effects or possible complications after trauma:

- Pulp obliteration (no RCT necessary because expression of a healing process)
- Pulp necrosis (RCT necessary)
- Pulpitic symptoms (RCT necessary)
- Internal granuloma (RCT necessary)
- Infection-related resorption (immediate RCT necessary because of rapid progression)
- Replacement resorption with new bone formation and subsequent ankylosis of the tooth (especially critical at growing age because considerable loss of space can ensue; treatment options are very limited in the event of ankylosis)
- Other: root growth abruptly ends, formation of a phantom root, or gingival recession

The focus is always on tooth preservation, at least until a time when satisfactory, ongoing treatment is possible.

TREATING CHILDREN IN PAIN

Treating children in pain is one of the greatest challenges in everyday practice. The child's compliance is sometimes greatly impaired, and it is not usually possible to take a precise pain history. We cannot resort to customary diagnostic criteria such as pulp and percussion tests in most cases, especially in infants. In addition, the patient's attendance is usually unplanned. Acute pain treatment is often a compromise, but there is nothing wrong with that provided further treatment is carried out, the parents are informed about the nature of the treatment, and, of course, the treatment alleviates the pain and is performed correctly.

Apart from trauma, the classic situation is an aching primary tooth, hence pulpitic symptoms or "swollen cheek," which means odontogenic infections caused by caries.[90] As well as performing basic diagnostics (intraoral and extraoral examination and radiographs), the clinician obviously needs to treat causally within the scope of what is possible. Pains that are caused by eruption of teeth, aphthae, or gingivitis require a purely symptomatic treatment. Teeth with pulpitic symptoms or apical periodontitis need to be treated causally.

In any event, this stressful visit to the dentist must be kept as short as possible for the child, which means avoiding long waiting times. It is important to reassure the parents and respond to the child with empathy, as this also has a demonstrable pain-relieving effect.[91] One should always bear in mind that, as well as the causal therapy, it is about ensuring the cooperation of the young patient,[90] because treatment very often cannot be completed in a single session.

It may become necessary to prescribe analgesics, depending on the findings. Acetaminophen or ibuprofen can be considered for the purpose, the latter being preferred because of its longer duration of action, lower toxicity, and wider therapeutic range.[91] Ibuprofen is available as an oral suspension, and the dose is dependent on age and body weight (3×10 mg per kilogram body weight per day).

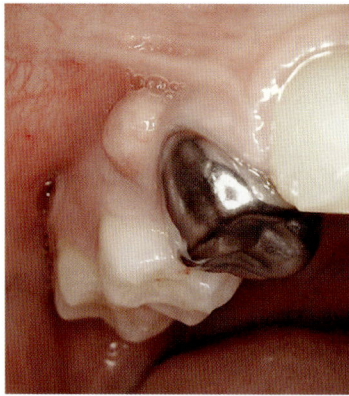

Fig 7-38 Fistulating primary tooth.

Pulpitic symptoms or "the aching primary tooth"

It is essential to ask how long the child has had the pain. As soon as children are about 3 years old, they are able to say where the pain is located. It is important to take a precise pain history to find out the inflammatory state of the primary tooth pulp, because this determines the nature of further treatment.[90] If the pain has occurred for the first time, if it is stimulus-dependent, and if the tooth shows no interradicular abnormalities on radiographs (reversible pulpitis), there is a possibility of preserving the tooth with a pulpotomy. If this is not possible in the context of acute treatment, caries should at least be excavated, and a temporary filling should be placed. If compliance is inadequate for anesthesia, a compromise solution would be partial caries excavation followed by placement of a temporary filling made of zinc oxide eugenol cement (the prerequisite is no hypersensitivity to eugenol). Taking into account the state of the residual dentition and the patient's compliance, either the child should be referred to a specialist (eg, no compliance, significant caries), or a prompt appointment should be arranged for definitive treatment with anesthesia (eg, pulpotomy and crown).

If the symptoms have lasted some time in the form of prolonged pain or if the pain can be provoked by pressure, for instance, and there is no interradicular radiolucency, the tooth can be preserved by means of a pulpectomy (irreversible pulpitis). If this fails due to the child's lack of compliance and/or if loosening, swelling, interradicular radiolucency, and/or a fistula is present (Fig 7-38), this suggests an advanced inflammatory process. In these cases, tooth preservation is not possible, and preference must be given to extraction.

In relation to pulpitic primary teeth, a common procedure is often to trephine and leave the tooth open. In the author's opinion, this approach cannot be recommended for various reasons (see below). Bücher et al write: "Trephination of pulpitic primary teeth is rarely an option because preference should be given to extraction if compliance is adequate and an effective local anesthetic can be applied."[90]

Dentogenic infections or "swollen cheeks"

In the presence of dentogenic abscesses, it is essential to assess how bad the finding is. If the child's general condition is impaired, if the child has a fever or is immunosuppressed, and if the course is progressive, in-patient admission with intravenous antibiotic administration is indicated. However, this is rarely the case.

If this is primarily a healthy child without fever, either the tooth responsible must be extracted straight away, or the acute inflammation should first be converted into a chronic state. Immediate extraction is advantageous for several reasons: a process is created via the extraction wound, the clinician is not dependent on the parents' reliability for a follow-up visit, and no renewed intervention is necessary. A problematic aspect of this approach is adequate anesthesia, which should not be carried out in the inflamed region. This point sometimes proves difficult in practice and in terms of technical compliance, necessitating a compromise treatment. This consists of trephination, leaving the affected tooth open, and symptom-based analgesia with concurrent antibiotic use.[91]

In the author's opinion, this method has a few drawbacks. First, trephination must be performed, which is often problematic for children. Even if the primary tooth is necrotic and exhibits no sensitivity, trephination is often unpleasant due to the pressure and vibration, while compliance is limited because of the pain. Second, a secondary treatment *must* be performed on the tooth even though it is currently still causing the child pain and still shows interradicular inflammation in 1 week's time, which might impede the depth of anesthesia. This means we are also dependent on the parents' reliability, who absolutely must attend the second appointment. We also have to hope that the child will be sufficiently cooperative in the second session. Below are the possible failures of this compromise treatment, which particularly specialists will encounter frequently in everyday practice:

- Unsatisfactory compliance at the extraction appointment
- Persistence of the trephined primary teeth
- Recurrent abscess formation
- Fracture of the trephined primary teeth
- Difficult extraction of primary teeth left open for a long time
- Structural anomalies and/or ectopic eruption of the permanent successors (Fig 7-39)

Dental practitioners should be mindful of these drawbacks in their pain management. If the parents are very unreliable, for instance, it might actually be preferable to remove the tooth concerned straight away. The advantage of this approach is that primary teeth that are responsible for an abscess no longer have any interradicular or periapical bone attachment and are usually very easy and unproblematic to remove under normal circumstances. Some practitioners prefer pulpectomy for severely inflamed and/or abscess-causing primary teeth rather than extraction. According to the author, this approach should be considered very carefully with regard to the healthy development of the successive tooth. Furthermore, the approach does not seem suitable for general dental practice.

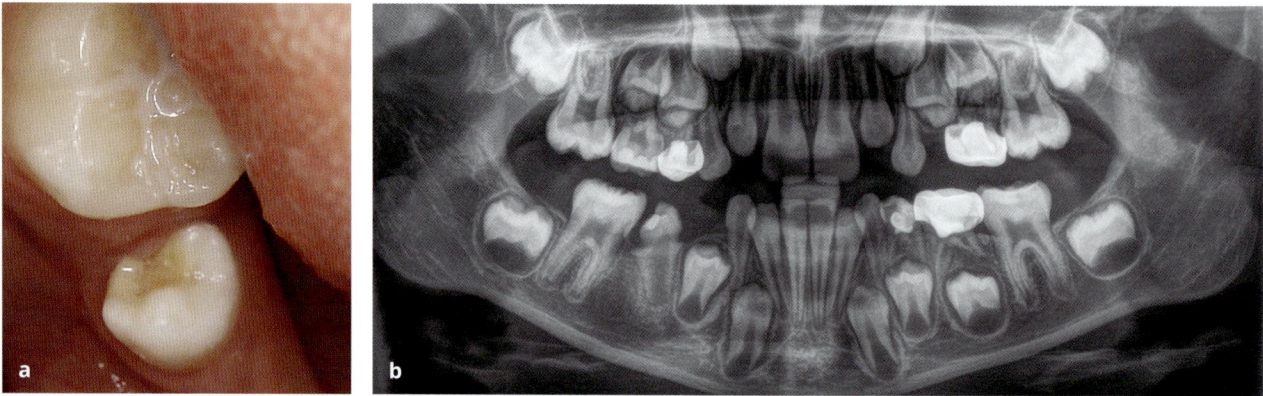

Fig 7-39 *(a and b)* Ectopic eruption of the permanent second premolar with occlusal enamel anomaly after preceding untreated apical periodontitis of a primary molar.

INCISION IN CHILDREN – YES OR NO?

Bücher et al write: "Only for fluctuating and purulent processes does incision appear to be the procedure of choice for providing rapid and effective relief. However, this requires local anesthesia and good cooperation. If there is edematous infiltration of the surrounding soft tissue, as encountered more commonly in children, incision is not expedient because an encapsulated inflammatory process is not present. Against the background of possible traumatization of the child, priority should be given to antibiotic treatment in these cases."[90]

Tip: An incision in the primary dentition can often be avoided by draining pus through the periodontal space. Because of the loose junctional epithelium, it is often enough to massage the swollen vestibulum and thereby ensure vestibular drainage of pus from the affected tooth. Parents can also carry out this measure at home in the acute phase. Widening the periodontal space with a spatula is often enough to achieve drainage.

Simple administration of antibiotics and analgesics without any pus-draining measures and/or causal therapy is contraindicated. Figure 7-40 presents the factors that should be considered in decision-making when selecting the right therapeutic measures.[90]

Urgency	High		Moderate			
	(eg, subcutaneous abscess, multiple trauma)	(eg, odontogenic abscess, complex anterior dental trauma)	(eg, pulpitis, acute apical periodontitis or swelling/inflammatory infiltrate, anterior dental trauma)			
Procedure can be performed under local anesthesia	No	Yes	No		Yes	
Expectation of child's cooperation	Negative	Negative / Positive	Negative / Positive		Negative / Positive	
Need for antibiotic therapy/analgesia	Without influence on the procedure	If required, intravenously or orally perioperatively	If required, orally preoperatively			
Treatment	Emergency procedure under sedation/endotracheal anesthesia	Emergency procedure under LA	Elective procedure under LA	Elective procedure under sedation/endotracheal anesthesia	Elective procedure under LA	

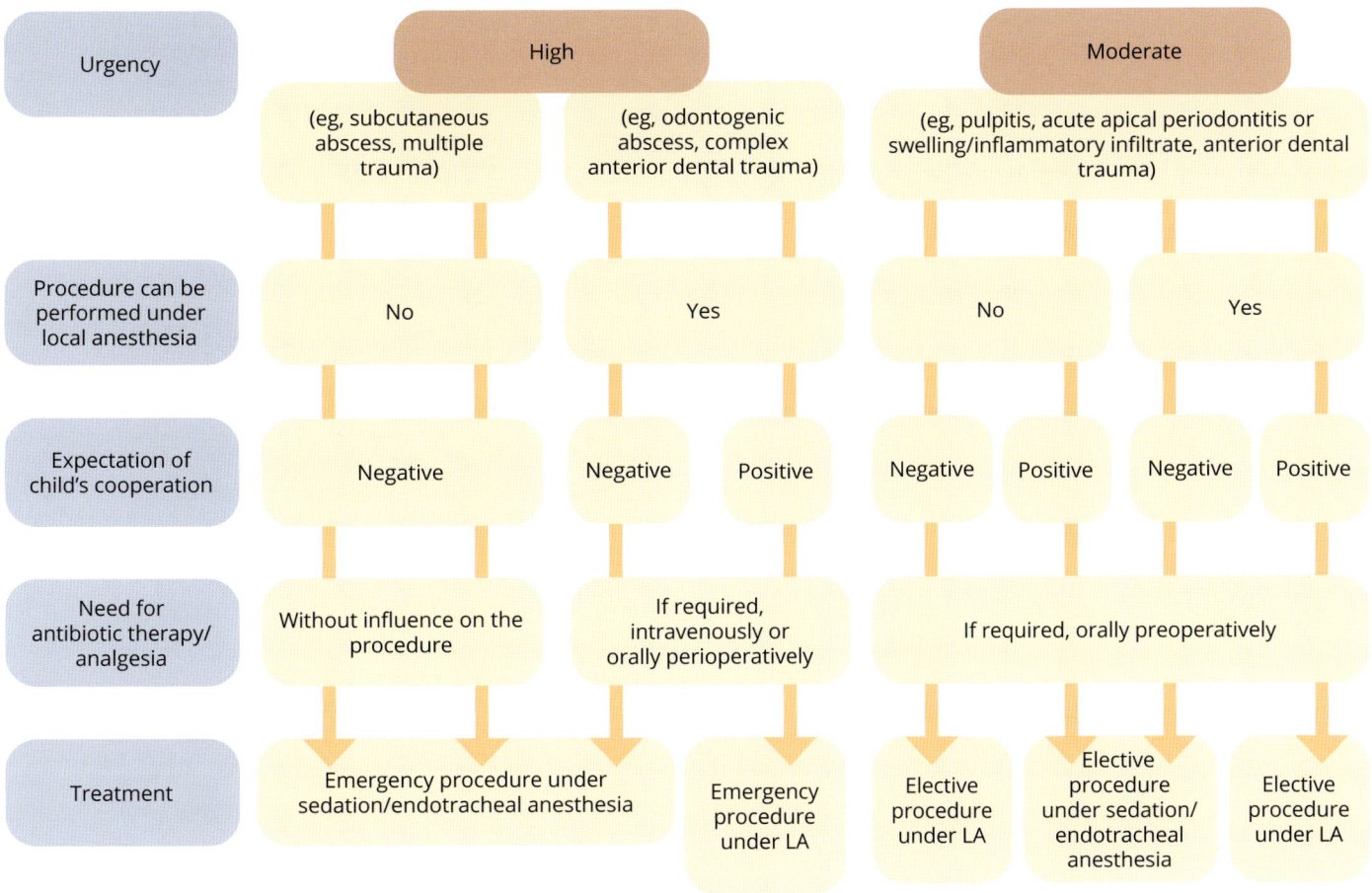

Fig 7-40 Factors that should be involved when choosing the appropriate therapeutic measures for pain management. LA, local anesthesia. (Data from Bücher et al.[90])

ANTIBIOTIC USE IN CHILDREN

As in adults, antibiotics should only be given to children in justified exceptional cases. Antibiotics are not indicated and are inadvisable as pain therapy, for instance in acute pulpitis.[92] Similarly, viral conditions do not require antibiotics, unless secondary bacterial colonization is suspected.[93] Antibiotic use is not necessary in the case of fistulae or after immediate removal of the affected tooth.[90] According to the guidelines of the European Academy of Paediatric Dentistry (EAPD), the following are the indications for additional antibiotic therapy in children, of course alongside elimination/treatment of the primary cause:

- Endocarditis prophylaxis
- Acute, very quickly progressing infections with moderate swelling and severe pain or accompanying fever
- Dentogenic infections in immunosuppressed children
- Subcutaneous abscesses, for which immediate in-patient referral is advisable
- Osteomyelitis
- Severe trauma and replantation of teeth
- Aggressive periodontitis in children and adolescents

The duration of treatment is given as 3 to 7 days.[94]

The following are effective antibiotics for the management of dental infections: penicillin, clindamycin, erythromycin, cephalosporin, metronidazole, and tetracycline. These antibiotics are effective against streptococci (except metronidazole) and anaerobes.

The EAPD guidelines on antibiotic use in children state the following: Despite its relatively narrow spectrum of action, phenoxymethylpenicillin (penicillin V) is the antibiotic of choice for dentogenic infections. The Paul Ehrlich Society also advises using penicillin V in children under 6 years.[90,91] Clindamycin can be used for patients with penicillin allergies. The use of amoxicillin in combination with clavulanic acid is suitable for school-age children and adolescents.[90] Amoxicillin should be used in the context of endocarditis prophylaxis.[94] Tetracyclines are the antibiotic of choice in the case of trauma, although the patient's age should be borne in mind in view of the possibility of tetracycline discoloration (see below).

Because it takes at least 24 hours for the onset of pain reduction, it is advisable to prescribe an analgesic additionally for the first 2 days,[90] preferably ibuprofen (3 × 10 mg per kilogram body weight per day).

The common antibiotics are available as oral suspensions or granules, making administration easier, especially in children. The most popular antibiotics are presented below with dosage examples for a typical selected compound in the form of oral suspension or granules. The following recommendations are taken from the AAPD document, Useful Medications For Oral Conditions.[95] It states: "Decisions about drug therapy must be based upon the independent judgment of the clinician, changing drug information, and evolving health care practices." The following recommendations should therefore only be seen as indications that must be examined by the clinician for each case and patient.

Penicillin V potassium[95]

Caution: The practitioner should use penicillin cautiously in patients with renal impairment or history of seizures. Anaphylactic reactions have been demonstrated in patients receiving penicillin, most notably those with a history of β-lactam hypersensitivity, sensitivity to multiple allergens, or prior immunoglobulin E–mediated reactions (eg, angioedema, urticaria, anaphylaxis). This antibiotic should be taken on an empty stomach because it is degraded by acid and enzyme activity in the stomach associated with ingestion of food.

Forms: Liquid, tablet

Usual oral dosage:

- *Children <12 years:* 25–50 mg/kg/day in divided doses every 6–8 hours (maximum 3 g/day)
- *Children ≥12 years and adults:* 250–500 mg every 6–8 hours

Amoxicillin clavulanate potassium[95]

Use the lowest dose of clavulanate combined with amoxicillin available to decrease gastrointestinal adverse drug events.

Forms: Suspension, chewable tablet, tablet

Usual oral dosage:

- *Children >3 months of age up to 40 kg:* 25–45 mg/kg/day in doses divided every 12 hours (maximum single dose 875 mg; prescribe suspension or chewable tablet due to clavulanic acid component)
- *Children >40 kg and adults:* 500–875 mg every 12 hours (prescribe tablet)

Amoxicillin[95]

Forms: Suspension, chewable tablet, tablet, capsule

Usual oral dosage:

- *Infants >3 months, children, and adolescents <40 kg:* 20–40 mg/kg/day in divided doses every 8 hours (maximum 500 mg/dose) *OR* 25–45 mg/kg/day in divided doses every 12 hours (maximum 875 mg/dose)
- *Adolescents and adults:* 250–500 mg every 8 hours *OR* 500–875 mg every 12 hours
- *Endocarditis prophylaxis:* 50 mg/kg (maximum 2 g) 30–60 minutes before procedure

Clindamycin[95]

Note: This is one of two options for patients with Type I allergic reactions to penicillin and/ or cephalosporin antibiotics. This antibiotic is effective for infections (eg, abscesses) with gram-positive aerobic bacteria and gram-positive or gram-negative anaerobic bacteria.

Forms: Suspension, capsule, injectable

Usual oral dosage:

- *Children:* 8–20 mg/kg/day in three to four divided doses as hydrochloride *OR* 8–25 mg/ kg/day in three to four divided doses as palmitate
- *Adults:* 150–450 mg every 6 hours (maximum 1.8 g/day)
- *Endocarditis prophylaxis:* 20 mg/kg (maximum 600 mg) 30–60 minutes before procedure

Doxycycline[95]

Especially in severe trauma cases (intrusion, avulsion, severe lateral dislocation), administration of doxycycline (tetracycline) is recommended because it has antibacterial and antiresorptive properties. For children under 8 years, administration of doxycycline is not recommended because the crowns are not yet mineralized and can sustain tetracycline discoloration. However, Weiger et al write that such discoloration is rather unlikely following short-term administration for 7 days.[85] Pregnant women should not take doxycycline either.

Forms: Suspension, tablet, delayed-release tablet, capsule, injectable

Usual oral dosage for necrotizing ulcerative gingivitis:

- *Children >8 years who weigh <45 kg:* 2.2 mg/kg every 12 hours on day 1, then 2.2 mg/kg once/day; for severe infections, 2.2 mg/kg every 12 hours until infection resolves
- *Children >8 years who weigh >45 kg and adults:* 100 mg every 12 hours on day 1, then 100 mg once/day; for severe infections, 100 mg every 12 hours until infection resolve

Usual oral dosage for avulsion, intrusion, or severe lateral dislocation (>5 mm) of permanent teeth:

- *Children (8 years and older) below 50 kg:* 4 mg/kg on the first day, then 2 mg/kg/day for 7 days
- *Adolescents and adults over 50 kg:* 200 mg on the first day, then 100 mg/day for 7 days

OVERVIEW OF ANTIBIOTIC USE

Unfortunately, medicinal treatment of children is frequently incorrect or inadequate.[96] In view of growing antibiotic resistance, it is absolutely essential for us as practitioners to use antibiotics as restrictively as possible but, if they are necessary, definitely use high-enough doses and for an appropriate period of time. It is imperative to explain to parents that the symptoms disappearing does not justify stopping the medication before the agreed time. Table 7-4 provides a summary and quick reference on the dosage regimens for the most common antibiotics. Detailed dosage recommendations for possible examples of these medications can be found above in the relevant text.

TABLE 7-4 Dosage of typical antibiotics[90]

Active substance	Dosage (oral)	Indication
Penicillin V potassium	*Children <12 years:* 25–50 mg/kg/day in divided doses every 6–8 hours (maximum 3 g/day) *Children >12 years and adults:* 250–500 mg every 6–8 hours	Odontogenic infections (eg, submucous abscess, acute apical periodontitis, provided tooth removal is possible); children < 6 years
Amoxicillin clavulanate potassium	*Children >3 months of age up to 40 kg:* 25–45 mg/kg/day in doses divided every 12 hours (maximum single dose 875 mg; prescribe suspension or chewable tablet due to clavulanic acid component) *Children >40 kg and adults:* 500–875 mg every 12 hours (prescribe tablet)	
Amoxicillin	*Infants >3 months, children, and adolescents <40 kg:* 20–40 mg/kg/day in divided doses every 8 hours (maximum 500 mg/dose) *OR* 25–45 mg/kg/day in divided doses every 12 hours (maximum 875 mg/dose)	Odontogenic infections previously treated with antibiotic; odontogenic abscesses; children > 6 years; adolescents
Clindamycin	*Children:* 8–20 mg/kg/day in three to four divided doses as hydrochloride *OR* 8–25 mg/kg/day in three to four divided doses as palmitate	In case of penicillin/amoxicillin intolerance

SEDATION

Benzodiazepines

Sedation possibilities with medication, such as midazolam, are always considered if compliance is inadequate for necessary treatment but the findings do not justify treatment under endotracheal anesthesia. In the author's opinion, benzodiazepines should always be administered to children in the presence of an experienced anesthetist because only such a specialist can dose the relevant medication high enough to avoid a paradoxical reaction and at the same time manage any complications safely. Midazolam is suitable for single-tooth extractions (eg, after trauma), for instance, or for manageable treatments of children who are still too young for nitrous oxide to be used. As a result of the anterograde amnesia that occurs, children later know nothing about the dental treatment, which can certainly be advantageous for further desensitization. Someone who cannot safely control any complications that may arise during a sedation should NOT carry out this procedure on their own. Do not be a hero on this topic. It is strongly advisable to find a dental anesthesiologist who will come to the office, do the sedation, and monitor the child. Using nitrous oxide is by far a better and safer method to use.

Nitrous oxide

Nitrous oxide (eg, "laughing gas") is a wonderful form of sedation in pediatric dentistry and can help to avoid remedial work under anesthesia. Nitrous oxide can bridge the gap between local anesthesia and the need for general anesthesia. Children who reliably breathe through their nose with their mouth open and tolerate a nasal mask well can be treated with laughing gas. This is usually the case for children ages 4 to 5 years. Nitrous oxide has several advantages: It acts quickly, it preserves protective reflexes, the patient remains responsive, and there are no paradoxical reactions and rarely any side effects. Laughing gas can be used for patients in the American Society of Anesthesiologists (ASA) classes 1 and 2 (physical status classification system). The only real contraindications to the use of nitrous oxide are poor compliance, impaired nasal breathing, chronic obstructive pulmonary diseases, vitamin B12 deficiency (caution with children on a vegan diet), bowel obstruction, existing or recent middle ear infection, and administration of nitrous oxide less than 4 days previously.[97]

Some anesthetists regard nitrous oxide use by a dentist as questionable; however, the AAPD considers it a safe and effective technique to reduce anxiety, produce analgesia, and enhance effective communication between a patient and health care provider.[98] It is certainly the case that sedation with laughing gas, which is a mixture of oxygen and nitrous oxide, is the safest form of outpatient sedation of children. No fatalities connected with nitrous oxide sedation have been documented, and an overdose can be readily managed by the dentist. Furthermore, modern devices will only permit dosing that always remains within set limits, beyond which a serious risk to health might be possible. Remedial work can be performed quadrant by quadrant in children with the aid of nitrous oxide, and the gag reflex can be kept well under control.

Hypnosis techniques can be combined with the use of nitrous oxide. Laughing gas masks can be wonderfully integrated into imaginative stories (eg, perhaps the mask can be a scuba diver's mask for the child to explore underwater). Additional anesthesia is crucial because you will not achieve pain elimination with the usual dosages in a dental practice. In addition, vital functions should be monitored with a pulse oximeter, and it goes without saying that dentists and dental assistants require special further training in this field, ideally including practical exercises.

Endotracheal anesthesia

The treatment of infants/children under endotracheal anesthesia should be carried out by a specialist. Especially remedial work on ECC, which mainly affects very young patients and can sometimes be very complex and time-consuming, should only be performed by experienced practitioners. Unfortunately, the availability of certified pediatric dentists is inadequate in many, largely rural, regions so that children requiring extensive remedial work are not uncommonly referred to surgical practices because they have facilities for general anesthesia. For this reason, a few basic points about treating children under endotracheal anesthesia are briefly discussed below.

• Endotracheal anesthesia is not indicated if the amount of treatment involved is minimal (eg, a few teeth or only in one affected quadrant). In these cases, other treatment alternatives should be chosen (eg, arresting caries by methods such as application of fluorides or SDF, Hall technique, fillings, or sedation if compliance is lacking). Endotracheal anesthesia carries a considerable risk, especially in very small children, and it should thus be used restrictively. It is the anesthetic method of choice if treatment is required in all four quadrants or if several extractions or endodontic treatments are indicated and compliance is poor.

- Before carrying out endotracheal anesthesia, the dentist must identify the reasons for the greatly increased caries activity and should work with the parents on modifying the child's behavior. It makes no sense to expose children to the risk of endotracheal anesthesia and then leave the prevailing conditions unchanged. The parents need to be informed, made aware, guided, motivated, and remotivated. This is not done in one or two sessions; it takes persistence. There are repeatedly cases where children have considerable need for treatment again after 2 or 3 years, which is also very frustrating for the dentist. Furthermore, it must be made clear to parents that there is always a risk associated with endotracheal anesthesia and repeated anesthesia should at all events be avoided.

- Treatment involving endotracheal anesthesia should always be planned so it can be completed within the scheduled time (maximum 1 to 2 hours, depending on age). In the author's opinion, putting children under endotracheal anesthesia twice for remedial dental work is absolutely contraindicated.

- The nature of the remedial work is also guided by the conditions surrounding the patient. This means that children with very poor parental compliance need to be treated differently than children in whom a marked improvement is already evident beforehand. For patients with poor parental compliance, there is a risk that oral hygiene instructions will not be followed or certain dietary habits will not be modified after the anesthesia, and/or routine checkups with the dentist might not be kept. Microbial colonization on an SSC is less marked than on any filling material, and a tooth that has previously undergone pulpectomy is more likely to cause symptoms than an extracted tooth. Therefore, pulpectomies and time-consuming composite buildups should be avoided with such at-risk children. In this situation, remedial work should be done more radically and hence more sustainably with a lower chance of complications, which often means opting for extraction.

- In the author's opinion, temporary filling materials such as GIC or composite-reinforced GIC are absolutely contraindicated in cases involving endotracheal anesthesia.[99] Remedial work on a child under anesthesia places a great responsibility on the dentist and must be performed so that, as far as possible, a repeat procedure does not become necessary for the next 2 years. That is not the case with temporary filling materials in any circumstances. Composites and compomers can be used for posterior and anterior teeth. For these reasons, dentists who carry out endotracheal anesthesia must be familiar with the use of SSCs. Children needing remedial work under anesthesia have a very high risk of caries, which will not disappear merely through endotracheal anesthesia. The defects also tend not to be confined to the occlusal surfaces and are often close to the pulp; furthermore, the children's compliance is usually entirely unsatisfactory. During remedial work, the dentist should always question whether they can solve a potential future problem by standard treatment. If the answer is "no," the remediation must be done more radically. For example, for caries treatment with a residual dentin thickness of under 1 mm, a pulpotomy with crown restoration should preferably be performed, or, in the case of pulpotomies where safe hemostasis cannot be achieved, extraction should be preferred. No pulpectomy should be carried out in the molar region. The more uncertain the prognosis of the tooth, the more radical the remedial stage should be.

- Before any remedial work is performed under anesthesia, current dental radiographs must be available. Relying solely on clinical and pain diagnosis is not acceptable. If radiographs cannot be taken because of a lack of compliance with the equipment, they can be taken at the chairside if need be, provided the child is already sleeping. A preoperative panoramic radiograph may also be considered. In any case, the dentist needs to be informed about missing tooth germs, degrees of resorption, and the interradicular condition of the teeth. This is the only way to ensure the procedure is well planned and all the treatments can be completed within the scheduled time.

- It is important to give the parents rather more extensive information. If teeth have a questionable prognosis, the parents should always be told about extraction. If, after completion of the remedial work, fewer teeth have been removed than planned, it is easier for parents to accept than vice versa.

- Photographic documentation is always recommended before the start of remediation under endotracheal anesthesia.

- One week before the treatment appointment, the additional use of CHX mouthwash can be recommended for children who are already able to spit out reliably. In any event, the parents must maintain thorough oral hygiene with their children in order to minimize inflammation-related bleeding during the remedial work.

> **IMPORTANT NOTE**
> Before performing remedial work with endotracheal anesthesia in children, it is advisable for dentists to shadow and observe colleagues doing this kind of treatment. Many specialist pediatric practices offer such observation opportunities for colleagues.

Tips on simplifying treatment under endotracheal anesthesia

During treatment under endotracheal anesthesia, it is very helpful to have an extra assistant who can hand over items, do mixing, and document the procedure.

It is more convenient to have an anesthetist, who nasally intubates your patient, on site in the office. The space is very constricted during intubation through the throat. The tongue protruding a great deal is mainly a hindrance in the mandible. In this case, a good mouth prop (eg, a firmly lockable mouth gag) and the use of a rubber dam are good aids during remedial work. The dentist selects which side of the mouth to start with so that the anesthetist can fix the tube on the contralateral side. The rubber dam clamps are then fixed to the terminal teeth, usually the primary second molars. Subsequently, the slitted rubber dam already stretched over the frame is pulled over the clamps and fixed with wedges, or a piece of rubber dam is fixed approximally in the anterior dentition (split-dam technique). This method will definitely not create an absolute dry field as is possible with the single-hole technique, but the view and the dry field are far better than with cotton wool rolls alone. When preparing the rubber dam, dental assistants must make sure not to slit the rubber simply with scissors, as it will tear more easily. Two holes about 0.5 to 1 cm apart should be made, and only then should the space between be cut with scissors. To work more effectively, two curing lamps should be laid ready. Several fillings can even be cured at the same time under the rubber dam.

What is the optimal treatment procedure with endotracheal anesthesia?

In the case of endotracheal anesthesia, teeth should first be cleaned with CHX gel to address the gingivitis that usually exists as well as to remove any existing plaque. Fillings, pulpotomies/pulpectomies, and insertion of crowns should be performed next, and extractions should be performed at the end. Despite the endotracheal anesthetic, local anesthesia is recommended for extractions because it keeps children pain-free after waking and the usually highly inflamed extraction wounds will bleed less during the treatment.

What are the next steps after endotracheal anesthesia?

Children who have undergone remedial work under endotracheal anesthesia are and remain high-risk patients for the time being. This means that after remedial work, a checkup should be scheduled 1 to 2 days later, then again after a week, and subsequently the children should be involved in a 3-monthly recall system. These appointments, as well as fluoridation, should be used to improve children's compliance within the context of individual prophylaxis and also to remotivate the parents again and again.

OVERVIEW OF ENDOTRACHEAL ANESTHESIA

The treatment of children under endotracheal anesthesia belongs in the hands of practices specializing in pediatric dentistry. If that is not possible for various reasons, dentists who carry out treatments under anesthesia should undertake appropriate further training or shadowing. Remedial work under endotracheal anesthesia does not solve the problem; it merely eliminates a symptom. True to the motto "We restore, you maintain," children and parents need to be very closely monitored in such cases.

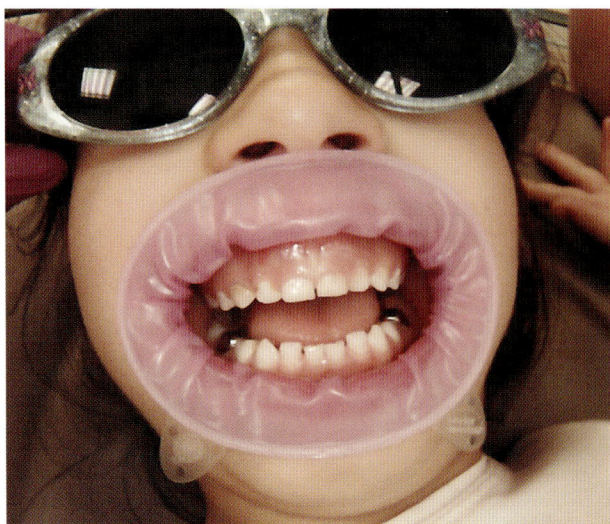

Fig 7-41 Patient with a mouth retractor as a treatment aid.

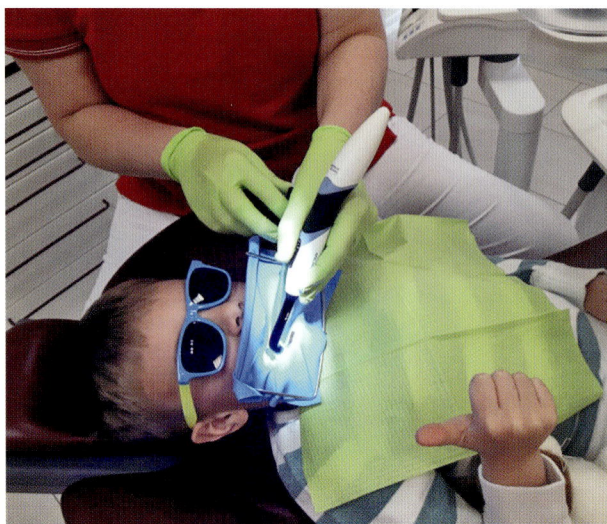

Fig 7-42 Relaxed treatment under rubber dam.

TREATMENT AIDS

Dry field

Creating a sufficiently dry field is often a difficult part of pediatric treatment. As well as classic cotton wool rolls, small dry tips inserted in the buccal area are very helpful. They are usually well tolerated by children, have good absorption capacity, and are easy to remove. It is also helpful to practice replacing cotton wool rolls in the mandible with the dental assistant. In this cotton wool roll replacement technique, the new roll already lies in position and simply has to be pressed downward while the dental assistant removes the wet roll lying underneath. A rubber dam or a mouth retractor can also be an excellent treatment aid. A mouth retractor makes mouth opening easier for children and effectively retracts the cheeks (Fig 7-41).

Before rubber dam placement in children, anesthesia or at least surface anesthesia can be administered beforehand. The clamp arms can slip under the equigingival cervical enamel bulge, which is painful. Positioning rubber dam clamps without surface anesthesia in the primary dentition is not recommended for this reason or only advisable with very cooperative children. Rubber dam clamps and serrated winged clamps are well suited to affix a rubber dam to the primary molars. It is advisable to cut the rubber dam after placement around the child's nose to make breathing a little easier. Another tip is to tie some floss on the lingual side of the clamp; in case it comes off, it can be removed more easily, and there is no chance that anything is swallowed or aspirated. Clamps that are suited well are no. 12A and 13A. The points of the clamp can always be blunted so it will not be so uncomfortable. Rubber dam placement can hugely simplify the treatment of a child (Fig 7-42). Understandably, many colleagues are reluctant to use this treatment aid because it takes some practice and because not every child will tolerate a rubber

Fig 7-43 Creating a dry field on an entire side of the jaw by the split-dam technique for remedial work under endotracheal anesthesia with intubation.

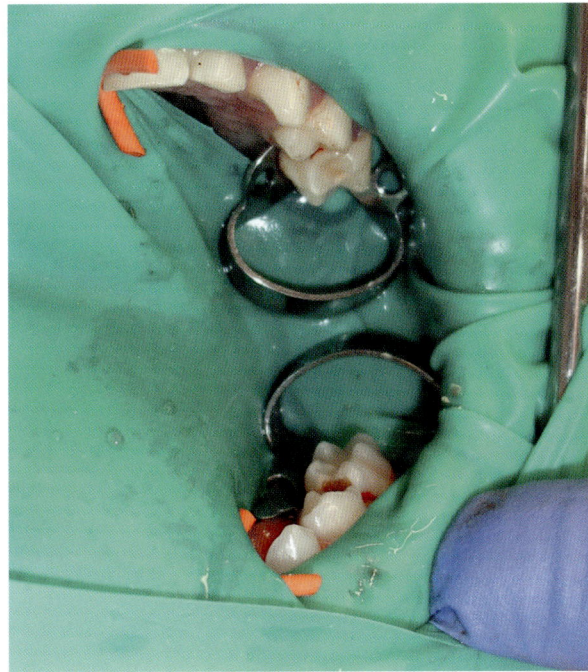

dam; children with restricted nasal breathing understandably have difficulties doing so. However, rubber dam use is obligatory with some measures (eg, pulpectomy).

The split-dam technique can be employed to simplify matters. Unlike puncturing the rubber dam in the single-hole technique for an individual tooth, the split-dam method involves splitting the rubber dam to accommodate several teeth. This is also suitable for treating class II defects. The clamp is first placed over the distalmost tooth of the teeth requiring treatment, and the rubber dam is then pulled by hand over the teeth lying mesial to that tooth. Wedges or a piece of cut-out rubber dam can be used to fix the dam in the interproximal space. In this way, remedial work can be done on groups of teeth or by quadrant, or a whole side of a jaw can be kept dry during the course of endotracheal anesthesia.

The quadrant-by-quadrant dry field created by the split-dam technique is obviously not quite as effective as the single-hole technique, but it does create good working conditions, especially for treatments performed under endotracheal anesthesia (Fig 7-43).

Mouth opening

Small, flexible mouth props have proved effective at keeping the mouth open in standard treatment. In the case of anesthesia, mouth props in metallic form are better to use because they take up less space in the oral cavity, they safely engage, and they are easily adjustable. A mouth retractor (available in junior sizes) is also a great help. Furthermore, Isolite (Zyris) is a special suction system that combines the bite wedge, suction, a light source, and certain aspiration protection.

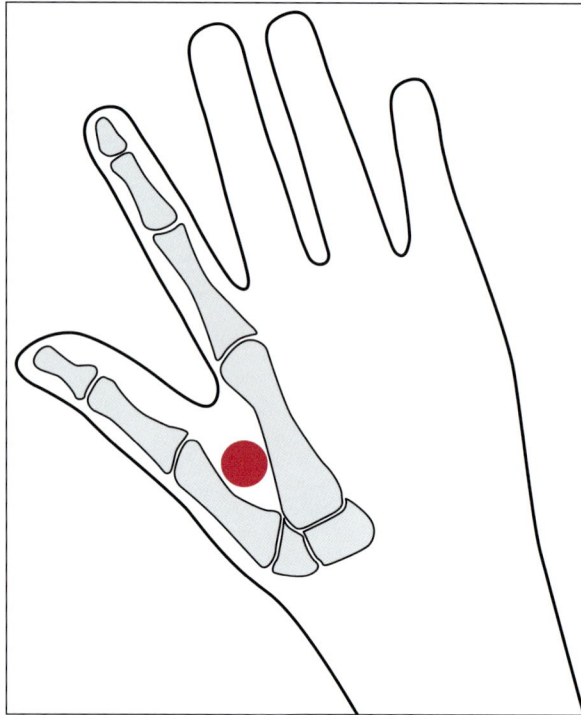

Fig 7-44 Location of acupressure point LI 4 for pain relief.

Acupressure

Acupressure can sometimes be helpful in pediatric dentistry for the patient and guardian, particularly very anxious mothers who cannot be separated from their child and who will likely disrupt the treatment unless you give them something useful to do. For instance, mothers can "hold hands" with their child while they massage the pressure point LI 4 (Fig 7-44). This can help relieve the child's pain and can distract and soothe the mother at the same time.

CASES THAT REQUIRE REFERRAL TO SPECIALISTS

When do you reach the limit of what is achievable in a general dentistry practice? This question cannot be answered in a single sentence because it primarily depends on the individual dentist and on the practice facilities (eg, sedation options, availability of materials such as crowns). Regardless of the complexity of the remedial work, the limit is reached whenever the remediation cannot be performed correctly, professionally, and conclusively. Many dentists reach their limitations with a primary tooth filling, others with an SSC, and still others with a child suffering from ECC, while on the other hand many general dentists carry out high-quality and even more complex treatments in children. Regardless of where one's own comfort zone with pediatric treatment ends, one thing is important: Do not carry out treatments that are not of the appropriate quality, only to treat patients temporarily without transferring them for definitive remedial care that is of the appropriate quality!

Of course, there will be compromise treatments in children, even by specialists. But the decisive difference is that the parents are informed about it, and other measures are taken to complete the treatment appropriately. Irrespective of where your treatment capabilities as a dentist end, your pediatric patients still deserve high-quality and especially definitive care. Whenever that is not possible, for whatever reason, the parents must be informed and referred to a specialist. This should be done before the child has undergone unnecessary treatment attempts and countless tears have been shed. The authenticity of acknowledging one's own limitations as a practitioner is not viewed negatively by parents. On the contrary, you will gain the confidence of your patients and also create long-term patient loyalty if the treatment is undertaken by a specialist in the meantime.

UNACCEPTABLE TREATMENT IN PEDIATRIC DENTISTRY
- Lengthy fixation of the child by the dentist or the practice team in order to perform treatments. Exceptions, for example, are brief holding by a parent for pain treatment that cannot be deferred (eg, extraction of a primary tooth severely damaged by trauma), during examination, or during necessary application of prophylactic preparations (eg, SDF, fluorides).
- Leaving inflamed or trephined primary teeth as "natural space maintainers."
- Toxavit (Lege Artis) and Depulpin (VOCO) dressings in primary teeth.
- Residual caries under temporary, nontight final fillings as a definitive restoration.

Unquestionably, not every pediatric treatment will go according to plan or have a satisfactory outcome. However, irrespective of how the treatment goes and how the child's or parents' compliance is gained, it is important to follow a few principles for quality-oriented dentistry and, above all, to provide information about the treatment. If a satisfactory and definitive treatment cannot be provided correctly with the facilities in your own practice, the patient must be referred to an appropriate specialist.

REFERENCES

1. Atzlinger F. Kinderhypnose in der Zahnheilkunde [thesis]. Budapest: Universität Budapest, Fakultät für Zahnmedizin, 2008. http://www.zahn1.at/service/downloads?file=files/assets/content/Download/DiplomarbeitKinderhypnoseinderZahnmedizinges.pdf. Accessed 26 August 2017.
2. Thumeyer A, Schlüter N. Prävention und noninvasive Therapie von (Initial-)Karies – eine besondere Herausforderung bei Kindern unter drei Jahren. ZMK 2016. Last updated 18 January 2016. https://www.zmk-aktuell.de/fachgebiete/kinderzahnheilkunde/story/ praevention-und-noninvasive-therapie-von-initial-karies--eine-besondere-herausforderung-bei-kindern-unter-drei-jahren_1404.html. Accessed 12 September 2017.

3. Gleissner C. Ergänzende Verfahren zur Erkennung des Kariesrisikos – eine Übersicht und kritische Betrachtung. ZMK. Last updated 2009. https://www.zmk-aktuell.de/fachgebiete/prophylaxe/story/ergaenzende-verfahren-zur-erkennung-des-kariesrisikos- -eine-Uebersicht-und-kritische-betrachtung_114.html. Accessed 24 August 2017.

4. Kühnisch J, et al. Kariesrisiko und Kariesaktivität. Quintessenz 2010;61:271–280.

5. Cariogram; Universitet Malmö. https://www.mah.se/fakulteter-och-omraden/Odontologiska-fakulteten/Avdelning-och-kansli/Cariologi/Cariogram/. Accessed 24 July 2018.

6. DAJ e.V. Grundsätze für Maßnahmen zur Förderung der Mundgesundheit im Rahmen der Gruppenprophylaxe nach § 21 SGB V, 2000. http://www.daj.de/fileadmin/user_upload/PDF_Downloads/grundsaetze.pdf. Accessed 30 October 2017.

7. Weber T. Memorix Zahnmedizin, ed 3. Stuttgart: Thieme, 2010.

8. Borutta A, Hellwig E, Kleeberg L. Kariesprophylaxe durch Intensivfluoridierung. ThiemeRefresher Zahnheilkunde 2011: R1-R16. https://www.cpgabaprofessional.de/content/ dam/cp-sites/oral-care/professional/de-de/professional-education/thieme-refresher.pdf. Accessed 29 August 2017.

9. Wegehaupt F. Remineralisation initialer Zahnhartsubstanzdefekte durch Fluoride und CPP-ACP? Oralprophylaxe Kinderzahnheilkunde 2017;39:38–44.

10. Krämer N. Wie wirksam ist Silber-Diamin-Fluorid? zm 2017;12. https://www.zm-online.de/archiv/2017/12/zahnmedizin/wie-wirksam-ist-silber-diamin-fluorid. Accessed 10 December 2018.

11. Sharma G, Puranik MP, Sowmya K. Approaches to arresting dental caries: An update. J Clin Diagn Res 2015;9:ZE09–ZE11.

12. Zhao IS, Mei ML, Burrow MF, Lo EC, Chu CH. Effect of silver diamine fluoride and potassium iodide treatment on secondary caries prevention and tooth discoloration in cervical glass ionomer cement restoration. Int J Mol Sci 2017;18(2):E340.

13. Smales R, Yip HK. The atraumatic restaurative treatment (ART) approach for primary teeth: Review of literature. Pediatr Dent 2000;22:294–298.

14. Fa Alvear B, Jew JA, Wong A, Young D. Silver modified atraumatic restaurative technique (SMART): An alternative caries prevention tool. Stoma Edu J 2016;3:18–24.

15. Gambon DL, Brand HS, Veerman EC. Dental erosion in the 21st century: What is happening to nutritional habits and lifestyle in our society? Br Dent J 2012;213:55–57.

16. Hedayati-Hajikand T, Lundberg U, Eldh C, Twetman S. Effect of probiotic chewing tablets on early childhood caries—A randomized controlled trial. BMC Oral Health 2015;15:112.

17. Villavicencio J, Villegas LM, Arango MC, Arias S, Triana F. Effects of a food enriched with probiotics on *Streptococcus mutans* and *Lactobacillus* spp. salivary counts in preschool children: A cluster randomized trial. J Appl Oral Sci 2018;26:e20170318.

18. Jørgensen MR, Castiblanco G, Twetman S, Keller MK. Prevention of caries with probiotic bacteria during early childhood. Promising but inconsistent finding. Am J Dent 2016;29:127–131.

19. Seminario-Amzez M, López-López J, Estrugo-Devesa A, Ayuso-Montero R, Jané-Salas E. Probiotics and oral health: A systematic review. Med Oral Patol Oral Cir Bucal 2017;22:e282–e288.

20. ZMK Sonderausgabe: Mikroinvasive Kariesbehandlung mit ICON. ZMK 2011;27. https:// www.zmk-aktuell.de/fachgebiete/zahnerhaltung/story/mikroinvasive-kariesbehandlung-mit-icon_515.html. Accessed 21 September 2017.

21. DMG: Icon Gebrauchsinformationen, 2015. https://de.dmg-dental.com/fileadmin/ user_upload/International/Instructions_for_use/GI_Icon_091909_int.pdf. Accessed 12 February 2020.

22. Ekstrand KR, Bakhshandeh A, Martignon S. Treatment of proximal superficial caries lesions on primary molar teeth with resin infiltration and fluoride varnish versus fluoride varnish only—Efficiency after 1 year. Caries Res 2010;44:41–46.

23. Ozgul BM, Orhan K, Oz FT. Micro-computed tomographic analysis of progression of artificial enamel lesions in primary and permanent teeth after resin infiltration. J Oral Sci 2015;57:177–183.

24. Turska-Szybka A, Gozdowski D, Mierzwińska-Nastalska E, Olczak-Kowalczyk D. Randomised clinical trial on resin infiltration and fluoride varnish vs fluoride varnish treatment only of smooth-surface early caries lesions in deciduous teeth. Oral Health Prev Dent 2016;14:485–491.

25. Twetman S. Strategies and measures for the reduction of ECC—What works? Vortrag bei der Jahrestagung der DGKIZ; Leipzig am 30.09.2017.

26. DGZMK: Leitlinie Fissuren- und Grübchenversiegelung; DGZMK, 2010; Autoren: Kühnisch J, Reichl FX, Hickel R, Heinrich-Weltzien R. http://www.dgzmk.de/uploads/tx_ szdgzmkdocuments/fissverslang.pdf. Accessed 1 October 2017.

27. Santamaria RM, Innes NP, Machiulskiene V, Evans DJ, Alkilzy M, Splieth CH. Acceptability of different caries management methods for primary molars in a RCT. Int J Paediatr Dent 2015;25:9–17.

28. Haghgoo R, Taleghani F. Comparison of periodontal ligament injection and inferior alveolar nerve block in mandibular primary molars pulpotomy: A randomized control trial. J Int Oral Health 2015;7:11–14.

29. Viergutz G, Hetzer G. Zahnärztlich-chirurgische Maßnahmen bei Kindern. Zahnmedizin update 2013;7:453–472.

30. Daubländer M, Kämmerer P. Lokalanästhesie in der Zahnmedizin; Sanofi Aventis; Berlin 2011.

31. DZW: Lokalanästhesie: Maximaldosis, Wirkstoff- und Adrenalingehalt ermitteln. https:// www.dzw. de/lokalanaesthesie-maximaldosis-wirkstoff-und-adrenalingehalt-ermitteln. Accessed 2 September 2017.

32. 3M ESPE: Fachinformation Lokalanästhetika, 2005. Accessed 2 September 2017.

33. Sanofi: Fachinformation Ultracain D-S, Ultracain D-S forte, 2015. Accessed 2 September 2017.

34. Splieth C. Invasive Kariestherapie im Milch- und Wechselgebiss; Fortbildungsveranstaltung der LZÄK Sachsen; Dresden, 11.04.–12.04.2014.

35. Randall R. Preformed metal crowns for primary and permanent molar teeth: Review of the literature. Pediatr Dent 2002;24:489–500.

36. DGZMK Leitlinie: Endodontie im Milchgebiss; DGZMK, 2011; Autoren: Kühnisch J, Heinrich-Weltzien R, Schäfer E. http://www.dgzmk.de/uploads/tx_szdgzmkdocuments/ 2011-03-25_Stellungnahme_ MZ-Endo_korrigiert.pdf. Accessed 2 July 2016.

37. Qvist V, Manscher E, Teglers PT. Resin-modified and conventional glass ionomer restorations in primary teeth: 8-year results. J Dent 2004;32:285–294.

38. Qvist V, Laurberg L, Poulsen A, Teglers PT. Class II restorations in primary teeth: 7-year study on three resin-modified glass ionomer cements and a compomer. Eur J Oral Sci 2004;112:188–196.

39. Qvist V, Poulsen A, Teglers PT, Mjör IA. The longevity of different restaurations in primary teeth. Int J Paediatr Dent 2010;20:1–7.

40. Pires CW, Pedrotti D, Lenzi TL, Soares FZM, Ziegelmann PK, Rocha RO. Is there a best conventional material for restoring posterior primary teeth? A network meta-analysis. Braz Oral Res 2018;32:e10.

41. Heuer L. Die Versorgung kariöser Milchmolarenläsionen mit Kompomer-Restaurationen und konfek-tionierten Kronen. Diss. Charité Berlin; Medizinische Fakultät 2016.

42. Krämer N, Frankenberger R. Füllungstherapie im Milchgebiss. Oralprophylaxe Kinderzahnheilkd 2004;26:78–84. http://zahnheilkunde.de/beitragpdf/pdf_1798.pdf. Accessed 6 September 2017.

43. AAPD Guideline of Restorative Dentistry, Reference Manual, 2016. http://www.aapd.org/media/ Policies_Guidelines/G_Restorative1.pdf. Accessed 5 September 2017.

44. Donmez SB, Turgut MD, Uysal S, et al. Randomized clinical trial of composite restorations in primary teeth: Effect of adhesive system after three years. Biomed Res Int 2016;5409393.

45. Yengopal V, Harneker SY, Patel N, Siegfried N. Dental fillings for the treatment of caries in the primary dentition. Cochrane Database Syst Rev 2009;15:CD004483.

46. Buerkle V, Kuehnisch J, Guelmann M, Hickel R. Restoration materials for primary molars—Results from a European survey. J Dent 2005;33:275–281.

47. Shaw AJ, Carrick T, McCabe JF. Fluoride release from glass-ionomer and compomer restorative materials. 6 months data. J Dent 1998;26:355–359.

48. Krämer N, Lohbauer U, Frankenberger R. Restorative materials in the primary dentition of poli-caries patients. Eur Arch Paediatr Dent 2007;1:29–35.

49. Schmalz G, Frankenberger R, Krämer N, Schwendicke F. Die Minimata-Konvention und Amalgam. Zahnärztliche Mitteilungen 2018;108:28–32.

50. zm online: Amalgamverbot für Kinder und Schwangere. zm online. Last updated 15 March 2017. Accessed 5 September 2017.

51. Shenker BJ, Maserejian NN, Zhang A, McKinlay S. Immune function effects of dental amalgam in children. J Am Dent Assoc 2008;139:1496–1505.

52. Bellinger DC, Trachtenberg F, Zhang A, Tavares M, Daniel D, McKinlay S. Dental amalgam and psycho-social status: The New England Children's Amalgam Trial. J Dent Res 2008;87:470–474.

53. Soncini JA, Maserejian NN, Trachtenberg F, Tavares M, Hayes C. The longevity of amalgam versus compomer/composite restorations in posterior primary and permanent teeth. J Am Dent Assoc 2007;138:763–772.

54. Lauenstein AS, Sieper A. Kronentherapie in der Kinderzahnheilkunde – Ein Überblick. Quintessenz 2015;11:1309–1315.

55. Innes NP, Evans, Stirrups DR. The Hall Technique; A randomized controlled clinical trial of a novel method of managing carious primary molars in general dental practice: Acceptability of the technique and outcomes at 23 months. BMC Oral Health 2007;7:18.

56. Ludwig KH, Fontana M, Vinson LA, Platt JA, Dean JA. The success of stainless steel crowns placed with the Hall technique—A retrospective study. J Am Dent Assoc 2014;145:1248–1253.

57. Santamaria R. Die Hall-Technik. zm 2017;107(13):28–30.

58. Evans D, Innes N. The Hall Technique—A minimal intervention, child centred approach to managing the carious primary molar. University of Dundee 2010. https://dentistry.dundee.ac.uk/files/3M_93C%20 HallTechGuide2191110.pdf. Accessed 4 September 2017.

59. Dobersch-Paulus S, Feierabend S. Kinderkronen step by step – Teil 1. ZMK 2009. https://www. zmk-aktuell.de/fachgebiete/kinderzahnheilkunde/story/kinderkronen-stepby-step--teil-1_62.html. Last updated 8 October 2009. Accessed 12 September 2017.

60. Dobersch-Paulus S, Feierabend S. Kinderkronen step by step – Teil 2. ZMK 2009. https://www. zmk-aktuell.de/fachgebiete/kinderzahnheilkunde/story/kinderkronen-stepby-step--teil-2_3861.html. Last updated 8 October 2009. Accessed 12 September 2017.

61. Dobersch-Paulus S, Feierabend S. Kinderkronen step by step – Teil 3. ZMK 2009. https://www. zmk-aktuell.de/fachgebiete/kinderzahnheilkunde/story/kinderkronen-stepby-step--teil-3_3862.html. Accessed 12 September 2017.

62. EZCrowns; website der Firma Sprig; Step-by-Step Instructions. https://sprigusa.com/posterior/. Accessed 3 August 2018.

63. AAPD: Guideline on Pulp Therapy for Primary and Immature Permanent Teeth; 2014. http://www. aapd.org/media/Policies_Guidelines/G_Pulp.pdf. Accessed 2 July 2017.

64. Gruythuysen RJ, van Strijp AJP, Wu M-K. Long-term survival of indirect pulp treatment performed in primary and permanent teeth with clinically diagnosed deep carious lesions. J Endod 2010;36:1490–1493.

65. Franzon R, Opdam NJ, Guimarães LF, et al. Randomized controlled clinical trial of the 24-months survival of composite resin restorations after one-step incomplete and complete excavation on primary teeth. J Dent 2015;43:1235–1241.

66. Heinrich-Weltzien R, Kühnisch J. Milchzahnendodontie. Zahnmedizin update 2007;2:145–168.

67. Zurn D, Seale NS. Light-cured calcium hydroxide vs formocresol in human primary molar pulpotomies: A randomized controlled trial. Pediatr Dent 2008;30:34–41.

68. Heinrich-Weltzien R, Kühnisch J. Endodontische Behandlungsmaßnahmen im Milchgebiss – Aktuelle Sichtweisen und Konsequenzen für die klinische Praxis. Oralprophylaxe Kinderzahnheilkd 2016;38:14–22.

69. Splieth C. Kinderzahnheilkunde in der Praxis. Berlin: Quintessenz, 2002.

70. DGZMK: Indikation und Gestaltung von Lückenhaltern nach vorzeitigem Milchzahnverlust, 2004. http://www.dgzmk.de/uploads/tx_szdgzmkdocuments/Indikation_und_ Gestaltung_von_Lueckenhaltern_nach_vorzeitigem_Milchzahnverlust-2004-07-01_1_.pdf. Accessed 14 October 2017.

71. Clausnitzer R. Lippen- und Zungenbändchen in der Kieferorthopädie; In: Furtenbach M. (Hrsg.) Das Zungenbändchen: die interdisziplinäre Lösung. Vienna: Praesens Verlag, 2007.

72. Hellwig E, Klimek J, Attin T. Einführung in die Zahnerhaltung – Prüfungswissen Kariologie, Endodontologie und Parodontologie. Köln: Dt. Zahnärzte Verlag, 2010.

73. Baxter R. Tongue Tied. Alabama Tongue-Tie Center, 2018.

74. Ghaheri B. Rethinking Tongue Tie Anatomy: Anterior vs. posterior is irrelevant. 2014. https://drghaheri.squarespace.com/s/Rethinking_TT_Anatomy.pdf. Accessed 5 January 2019.

75. Newman J. Breastfeeding – Empowering Parents. Independently published, July 2018.

76. Springer S. Das Leipziger Protokoll. In: Furtenbach M. (Hrsg.) Das Zungenbändchen: Die interdisziplinäre Lösung. Vienna: Praesens Verlag, 2007.

77. Bekes K, Krämer N, van Waes H, Steffen R. Das Würzburger MIH-Konzept: Teil 1. Der MIH-Treatment Need Index (MIH-TNI) - Ein neuer Index zur Befunderhebung und Therapieplanung bei Patienten mit Molaren-Inzisiven-Hypomineralisation (MIH). Oralprophylaxe Kinderzahnheilkd 2016;38:165–170.

78. Bekes K. Ätiologie und Therapie von MIH-Zähnen. ZWP online 2015. https://www.zwponline.info/fachgebiete/endodontologie/komplikationsmanagement/aetiologie-undtherapie-von-mih-zaehnen. Accessed 21 October 2017.

79. Discepolo K, Baker S. Adjuncts to traditional local anesthesia techniques in instance of hypomineralized teeth. N Y State Dent J 2011;77:22–27.

80. Lygidakis NA, Wong F, Jälevik B, Vierrou AM, Alaluusua S, Espelid I. Best clinical practice guidance for clinicians dealing with children presenting with Molar-Incisor-Hypomineralisation (MIH): An EAPD policy document. Eur Arch Paediatr Dent 2010;11:75–81.

81. Bekes K, Krämer N, van Waes H, Steffen R. Das Würzburger MIH-Konzept – Teil 2. Der Therapieplan. Oralprophylaxe Kinderzahnheilkd 2016;38:171–175.

REFERENCES

82. Steffen R, van Waes, H. Die Behandlung von Kindern mit Molaren-Inzisiven-Hypomineralisation. Eine Herausforderung bei der Shmerzkontrolle und Verhaltenssteuerung. Quintessenz 2011;62:1585–1592.

83. Viergutz G, Buske G. Parodontologie und Traumatologie im Milch- und Wechselgebiss; Fortbildungsveranstaltung der LZÄK Sachsen; Dresden; 16.05.–17.05.2014.

84. Schmoeckel J, Splieth C. Frontzahntrauma bei Kindern: Vorgehensweise in der Zahnarztpraxis. ZWP 2017; https://media.zwp-online.info/archiv/pub/gim/zwp/2017/ zwp0617/Schmoeckel_42.pdf. Accessed 20 October 2017.

85. AcciDent App. Autoren: Weiger R, Krastl G, Filippi A, Lienert N. Anbieter: YooApplicationsAG; Zahnunfallzentrum Universität Basel, 2014.

86. Kirschner H, Pohl Y, Filippi A, Ebeleseder K. Unfallverletzungen der Zähne – Ein Kompendium für Studium und Praxis. München: Elsevier Urban und Fischer, 2006.

87. Camilleri J. Staining potential of neo MTA Plus, MTA Plus, and biodentine used for pulpotomy procedures. J Endod 2015;41:1139–1145.

88. van Waes H, et al. Regenerative Endodontie. 2011; zwp-online. https://www.zwp-online. info/fachgebiete/endodontologie/fruehbehandlung/regenerative-endodontie. Accessed 20 January 2019.

89. Schneider E, Jepsen S, Dommisch H. Revaskularisierung avitaler Zähne. DZZ 2014;3(69):144–151.

90. Bücher K, et al. Schmerz- und Notfallbehandlung in der Kinderzahnheilkunde. Quintessenz 2016;67:411–420.

91. Heinrich-Weltzien R, Wagner Y. Schmerzbehandlung im Kindesalter. Spitta 2017; https://www.spitta. de/fachthemen/zahnmedizin/kinderzahnheilkunde/story/schmerzbehandlung-im-kindesalter_90. html. Accessed 28 August 2018.

92. Peedikayil FC. Antibiotics: Use and misuse in pediatric dentistry. J Indian Soc Pedod Prev Dent 2011;29:282–287.

93. AAPD: Use of Antibiotic Therapy for Pediatric Dental Patients. https://www.aapd.org/research/ oral-health-policies--recommendations/use-of-antibiotic-therapy-for-pediatric-dental-patients/. Accessed 13 February 2020.

94. EAPD: Policy Document for the use of antibiotics in paediatric dentistry, 2002. http:// www.eapd.eu/ uploads/20A87CB2_file.pdf. Accessed 23 October 2017.

95. American Academy of Pediatric Dentistry. Useful Medications for Oral Conditions. https://www. aapd.org/globalassets/media/policies_guidelines/r_usefulmeds.pdf. Accessed 17 February 2020.

96. Howard RF. Current status of pain management in children. JAMA 2003;290:2464–2469.

97. von der Wense C. Lachgassedierung in der Kinderzahnheilkunde mit Tipps aus der Praxis; Fortbildungsveranstaltung von Lohmeier Praxisoptimierung; Göttingen, 24.10.2012.

98. AAPD. Use of Nitrous Oxide for Pediatric Dental Patients. https://www.aapd.org/media/Policies_ Guidelines/BP_UseofNitrous.pdf. Accessed 13 February 2020.

99. Krämer N. Narkose als letzte Option; Vortrag im Rahmen der Jahrestagung der DGKIZ; Leipzig, 29.09.2017.

EPILOGUE

"Popcorn is prepared in the same pot, in the same heat, and in the same oil, and yet the kernels do not pop at the same time. Don't compare your child to others. Their turn to pop is coming."

ANONYMOUS

Children as patients can be incredibly demanding and nerve-wracking, but they are also the most genuine and most grateful patients you can imagine. No "thank you" or warm handshake will leave you quite as happy as the melted bar of chocolate shyly conjured out of a child's backpack or the picture that a little patient has painted and proudly presents to you. Children can be the most trusting, most chatty, and most appreciative of patients. Our job as dentists, regardless of specialization, is to treat this target group entrusted to us as best we can and according to the latest knowledge available.

I hope this manual is both practical and helpful in allaying any fears or overcoming any inhibitions associated with pediatric treatment. At the same time, I hope readers will appreciate what responsibility we bear, especially when treating children. Not every colleague has to become a pediatric dentist, but all dentists are obliged to deal with or indeed treat their young patients and to make responsible decisions. If that means issuing a referral to a specialist, that is perfectly alright, and sometimes it is the best and most responsible choice for a little patient a practitioner can make. The great thing about our profession is that you never stop learning, so use each experience to learn. There are numerous possibilities like further training (check the AAPD website for more information), online education, shadowing an experienced colleague, textbooks, and more.

Last but not least, remember to have patience— with the screaming babies, sticky-handed schoolchildren, eye-rolling teenagers, and helicopter parents as well as with yourself. Like anything new, getting into pediatric dentistry involves a certain learning curve, and I wish you every success on your journey.

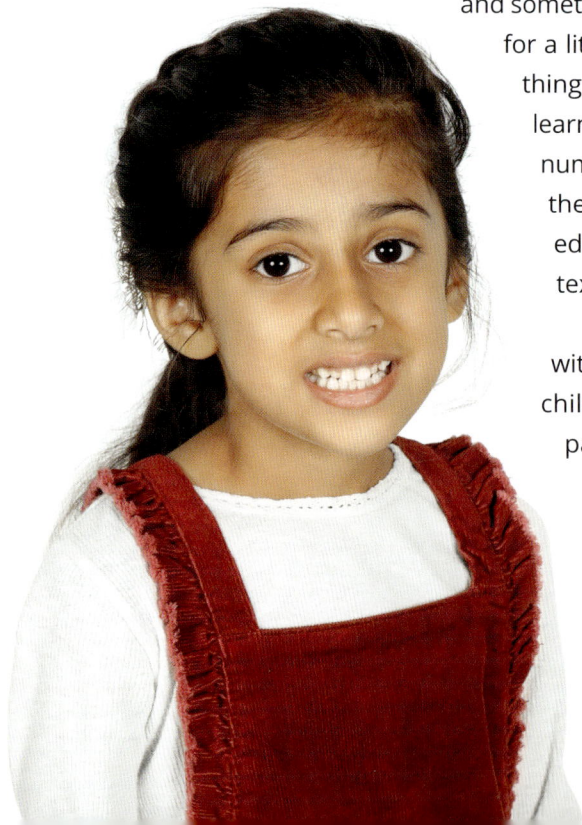

INDEX

Page references followed by "f" denote figures, "t" denote tables, and "b" denote boxes.

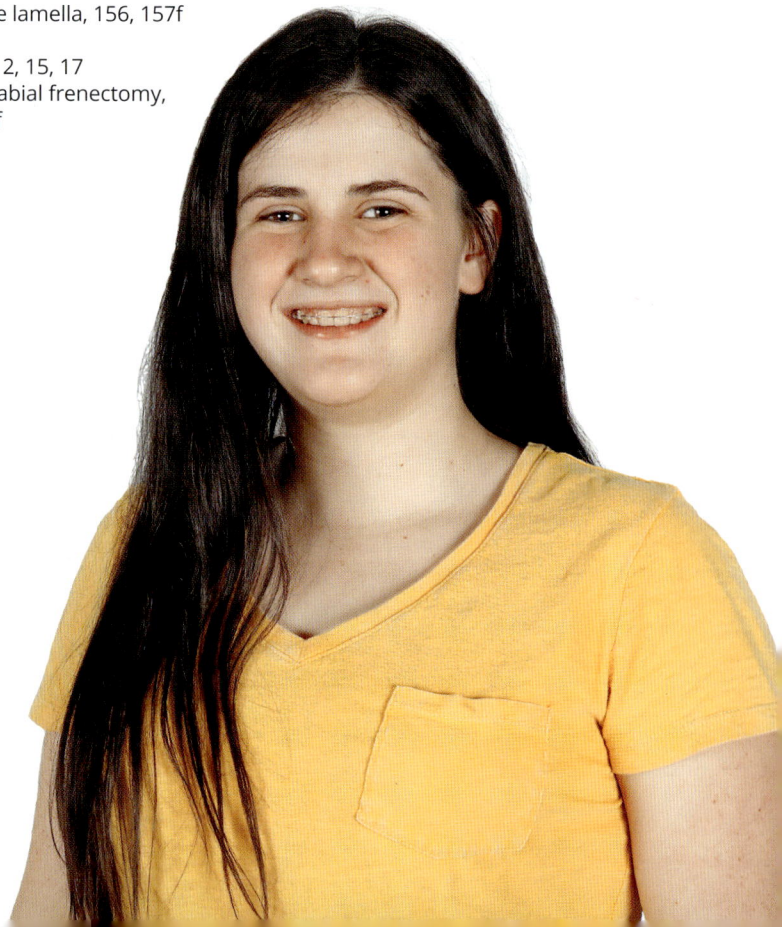